MW01292505

s.

To Jane Delano Brown
For forging the trail that we now travel together

CONTENTS

CONTRIBUTORS

Mariana Alonso-Fernández, Autonomous University of Madrid, Spain, is a Predoctoral Researcher in Psychology whose research focuses on promoting digital citizenship among young people and adults.

McCall Booth, Indiana University-Bloomington, United States, is a Ph.D. candidate who researches various social and psychological effects of media and digital technologies on relationships – from that of romantic partners to the parent–child dyad.

Sydney E. Brammer, Ph.D., University of North Florida, United States, is an Assistant Professor of Mass Communication who studies the impact of (emerging) media on users' identity through feminist lenses.

Enrica Bridgewater, University of Michigan, United States, is a Ph.D. candidate whose research examines media influences on ethnic/racial socialization for people of color.

Yuchi Anthony Chen, Ph.D., University of California-Irvine, United States, is a Postdoctoral Scholar who studies interpersonal and well-being implications of media and technologies, focusing on youth.

Angela Cooke-Jackson, Ph.D., California State University – Los Angeles, United States, is a Professor studying sexual health to promote the empowerment of young adults and gender minorities. She incorporates community-based participatory approaches that support communities' development of innovative sustainable changes.

Leticia Couto, Ph.D., DePaul University, United States, is an Assistant Professor in Public Relations and Advertising whose research focuses on message development and health behaviors.

Leah Dajches, Ph.D., New Mexico State University, United States, is an Assistant Professor whose research focuses on media effects in relation to marginalized audiences, identity, and adolescent development.

Rebecca Lin Densley, Ph.D., Trinity University, United States, is an Assistant Professor who researches the diverse ways media influence youth and how parents can play a role in mitigating negative media effects.

Christina V. Dodson, Ph.D., innovation Research and Training, United States, is a Research Scientist whose research explores media effects on health behaviors and the impact of media literacy education on the processing of media messages.

Manuel Gámez-Guadix, Ph.D., Autonomous University of Madrid, Spain, is an Associate Professor who researches internet problems like cyberbullying, problematic use, sexual and gender-based harassment, sexting, and online grooming, focusing on prevention from adolescence.

Rachell Hanebutt, Ph.D., United States, studies adolescent digital equity and well-being, leveraging teen-centric methods (i.e., CBPR, co-design) to advance the development and evaluation of digital well-being interventions via research–practice partnerships.

Stacey J.T. Hust, Ph.D., Washington State University, United States, is a Professor of Health Communication and Associate Dean of Faculty Affairs and College Operations. She studies how media influence adolescents' romantic and sexual lives.

C. J. Janssen, Washington State University, United States, is a master's student. Their research focuses on rural LGBTQ populations, gender studies, and media effects.

Arian Karimitar, Ph.D., Beth Israel Hospital, United States, is an Anthropologist and clinical researcher at a Harvard-affiliated medical research center. She studies how culture and society shape the processes of human cognition, emotion, perception, motivation, and mental health.

Hyelim Lee, Ph.D., Washington State University, United States, is an Assistant Professor whose research explores data-driven approaches and AI methods in communication strategies.

Yoon-Joo Lee, Ph.D., Washington State University, United States, is an Associate Professor who researches how consumers make sense of messages and on race and ethnicity issues in health communication. She also conducts research on corporate social responsibility, advertising, and public service announcements.

Charisse L'Pree Corsbie-Massay, Ph.D., Syracuse University, United States, is an Associate Professor who investigates the effect of media on how we think about ourselves and others and how we use media to affect how others think about us.

Chelly Maes, Ph.D., University of Leuven, Belgium, is a Postdoctoral Researcher whose work examines youth's digital media use, body image, and sexuality construction.

Marie-Louise Mares, Ph.D., University of Wisconsin–Madison, United States, is a Professor in the Department of Communication Arts at University of Wisconsin–Madison. She examines life-span development of media responses, recently focusing on identity, media, and family communication.

Jone Martínez-Bacaicoa, Autonomous University of Madrid, Spain, is a Predoctoral Researcher whose research focuses on the study of different forms of technology-facilitated sexual and gender-based abuse.

Rochelle R. Davidson Mhonde, Ph.D., George Mason University, United States, is Assistant Professor of Global and Community Health whose research includes examining help-seeking and communicative behaviors related to sexual trauma and other stigmatized health topics, particularly among minoritized communities.

Jessica Gall Myrick, Ph.D., Pennsylvania State University, United States, is the Donald P. Bellisario Professor of Health Communication. Her research examines the intersection of emotion and cognition in shaping audience responses to messages about health, science, and the environment.

Christina Griselda Nickerson, M.A., Washington State University, United States, is a Ph.D. candidate who studies the intersection of interpersonal-health communication and family communication within the context of adolescent reproductive health.

Rebecca Ortiz, Ph.D., Syracuse University, United States, is an Associate Professor in the S.I. Newhouse School of Public Communications whose research focuses on sexual health promotion, sexual violence prevention, and sexual media effects on adolescents and young adults.

Ron Price, M.A., Washington State University, United States, is a Ph.D. student who examines media's portrayals of minorities and their effects. He also studies the impact of cannabis marketing efforts.

Rachel E. Riggs, Ph.D., University of North Florida, United States, is an Assistant Professor who researches the role of media in encouraging adolescents' and emerging adults' disclosure of sexual assault and mental health problems.

Danielle Rosenscruggs, University of Michigan, United States, is a Ph.D. candidate in Developmental Psychology. Her research focuses on the impostor phenomenon in doctoral education and applied mitigation strategies.

Tracy M. Scull, Ph.D., innovation Research and Training, United States, is a Developmental Psychologist and Senior Research Scientist whose basic and applied research focuses on the promotion of health behaviors in childhood through emerging adulthood.

Jane Shawcroft, University of California – Davis, United States, is a Ph.D. student who researches how media and technology play a role in the social, mental, and emotional health of children and adolescents.

Jennifer Stevens Aubrey, Ph.D., University of Arizona, United States, is Professor of Communication who researches media effects on the mental well-being of youth.

Larissa Terán, Ph.D., Geena Davis Institute, United States, is Director of Media Research. She conducts research on media and marginalized groups.

Joy Wanja Muraya, Washington State University, United States, is a Ph.D. student who studies the development and evaluation of inclusive, effective health communication messages. Previously, she was a health and medical journalist in Kenya.

Laura Vandenbosch, Ph.D., University of Leuven, Belgium, is an Associate Professor whose core research is the relationship between media and well-being.

Joris Van Ouytsel, Ph.D., Arizona State University, United States, is an Assistant Professor whose work focuses on online risk behaviors.

L. Monique Ward, Ph.D., University of Michigan, United States, is Professor of Psychology whose research examines parental and media contributions to gender and sexual socialization for U.S. youth.

Jessica Fitts Willoughby, Ph.D., Washington State University, United States, is Lester M. Smith Distinguished Associate Professor in the Murrow College of Communication. She examines how media can be used to improve health attitudes and behaviors among adolescents.

Kun Yan, M.A., University of Arizona, United States, is a Ph.D. candidate who studies media effects, with a particular focus on social media and body image.

Carina M. Zelaya, Ph.D., University of Maryland, United States, is an Assistant Professor whose scholarship works to develop and evaluate evidence-based interventions – including mass media campaigns and messaging – that focus on disparities driven by social, racial, economical, and environmental factors.

FOREWORD

Jane D. Brown

As a young adolescent in the United States in the early 1960s, I remember watching movies to see what each person did after a kiss. I thought it would be embarrassing to have my face that close up to another person, especially a guy. I tried to replicate the eye makeup of the girls in *Seventeen* magazine and begged my mother for their skirt-and-sweater ensembles. But then bands like the Rolling Stones and the emerging women's liberation movement seduced me into the world of liberal politics, and sex, drugs, and rock "n" roll.

No more makeup, no more caring what I looked like. In college, I joined a cooperative that counseled young women about birth control and how to get an abortion in the few U.S. states where that was possible before *Roe vs. Wade* was decided in 1973. The media were helping me explore who I wanted to be. The images and messages I saw and heard were attractive but often incomplete and even contradictory (e.g., "Let's spend the night together" vs. "Going to the chapel and we're going to get married"). Today I know I was lucky I didn't suffer the negative consequences that were rarely portrayed or discussed.

As a young professor a decade later, I wondered how my experience of adolescence in the turbulent cultural moment of the late 1960s and early 1970s was similar or different for adolescents in the 1980s. The media world had changed dramatically, and my generation's "free love" mantra had contributed to a surge of teen pregnancies and sexually transmitted diseases. My students and I were intrigued by the debut of music videos, the audacity of Madonna's sexual imagery and persona, and the beginnings of Hip-Hop and rap. A new raft of magazines was targeting adolescents, selling perfect bodies and beauty products. Most teens now had televisions in their bedrooms, and movies had moved far beyond a chaste kiss in the sunset.

Our early studies of what are now called the "legacy media" (e.g., television, magazines) documented frequent sexual behavior in the media teens used, although the content was still rather benign by today's standards. As one media critic put it at the time, you were more likely to see a head cut off than a bare breast. We were still in an era of innuendo, kissing, and morning-after bedroom scenes. Just as now, however, "safe sex" – discussion or use of contraception in the context of loving, committed relationships – was extremely rare.

In 1993, Brad Greenberg, Nancy Buerkel-Rothfuss, and I co-edited *Media, Sex, and the Adolescent*. The chapters we co-authored with our students focused on the effects of soap operas, prime-time television, music videos, R-rated and mainstream films, and teen girl magazines. We could see even then that the use and effects of different kinds of media were influenced by access (TV in the bedroom or not), parental mediation, developmental stage (pre- or post-puberty), race, and gender.

A decade later (in 2002), I and two of my former students, Jeanne R. Steele and Kim Walsh-Childers, co-edited *Sexual Teens, Sexual Media: Investigating Media's Influence on Adolescent Sexuality*. The book's cover imagery of TV remote control devices and CDs (Compact Discs) in plastic cases is indicative that we were still in a different media world than today. The internet was discussed in only two of the 13 chapters.

In that book, we included more research about the different ways in which teens chose and interpreted media content and introduced the Media Practice Model. That model posited that teens' developing sense of themselves or identity affects what content they choose to pay attention to and how they respond to what they see or hear. We conceptualized the audience not as passive recipients but as active users who will be affected differently by the media content they choose.

That model of an active audience seems even more relevant now. Prime-time TV is an anachronism, as hundreds of channels and millions of videos are available on adolescents' cell phone screens. Only a few movies inspire teens to go to an actual theater these days, and print magazines are a thing of the past. Graphic pornography is a click away. A teen must be an active user to choose among this avalanche of sexual content.

In the early 2000s, some of the first longitudinal studies of media use and adolescents' sexual behavior were funded by the National Institutes of Health, the government agency responsible for biomedical and public health research in the United States. These studies were stimulated by a Congressional inquiry into the effects of sexual media content on vulnerable teen audiences. I and other social scientists argued that more research was needed, especially studies over time that could begin to disentangle causes and effects.

With the larger samples and new measures facilitated by subsequent multi-year large U.S. federal grants, several projects concluded that early adolescents' exposure to sexual content in the media is an important factor in earlier sexual activity (e.g., Brown et al., 2006). One of those studies even linked early exposure to sexual content to increased risk of teen pregnancy a few years later (Chandra et al., 2008).

Causality still remains an open question because the gold standard of randomized controlled trials is rarely possible in media studies. I think, however, that the consistent pattern of positive correlations in the existing well-conducted longitudinal studies is convincing that the sexual content in media does matter. Certainly, more longitudinal studies are merited as we continue to investigate the extent to which media are a causal factor in teens' sexual development.

If the rather tame legacy media made a difference in the early 2000s, what might we expect in this new anything-goes media world? With such remarkable access to all sorts of sexual content across many platforms, how do today's teens choose and absorb the media content with which they engage? What have we learned in the interim about the impact of the media on adolescents' sexuality?

I am glad to see these stellar scholars bringing us up to date by doing this important and often difficult research. As the editors discuss in an early chapter, it is not easy to gain access to minors to talk about sensitive issues. It also is not easy to accurately assess the amount and kind of media young people are using or to gauge the extent to which exposure affects sense of sexual self and sexual behavior.

These authors have met many of the challenges of this task. And we need more innovative research to delve even deeper into these important questions. I hope this book stimulates another generation of scholars to address the ways in which today's ubiquitous, explicit, and complicated sexual media world is processed and incorporated into young people's thinking and behavior.

Recent news reports suggest novel and disturbing possible effects that we didn't even contemplate a decade ago. In one U.S. middle school, the faces of girl students were superimposed on nude bodies using Artificial Intelligence programs and transmitted to other students (Healey, 2024). Another report suggested that adolescents are engaging in choking during intercourse because they've seen the dangerous practice in pornography (Orenstein, 2024).

The editors of this excellent compilation of recent research acknowledge that not only have media and media content changed, but cultural and political contexts are much different now than when we began asking these questions. Increased pushback about ideal body images, the advent of the #MeToo Movement, the broadening of definitions, and the politicalization of gender identities have changed significantly in the past two decades. Simultaneously, we are experiencing a dramatic shrinking of our rights to bodily autonomy. For the first time in 50 years, young people can't be sure that they will have access to an abortion if they need one, or even the right to use contraception. Gender-affirming care for adolescents is now forbidden in many U.S. states.

But some teens are using media to fight back. For example, youth activists in the United States used social media and the hashtag #FreeThePill to advocate for over-the-counter access to birth control pills; the U.S. Federal Food & Drug Administration (FDA) later approved the first birth control pill available without a prescription (Janfaza, 2023).

The chapters in this book offer novel ways of answering some of the important questions of this historical moment: How do modern media affect gender and sexual identities and subsequent relationships? How do teens interpret the sexual content they are choosing? Does readily accessible pornographic content affect teens' ideas about what is acceptable in sexual relationships? Do social media facilitate sexual violence?

I appreciate that the editors also have included a section on opportunities for advocacy and education. Media literacy education is more sophisticated than when we first suggested potential benefits several decades ago. Now we have evidence that the modern materials designed to educate young people about healthy ways to use media are effective.

The possibility of promoting sexual health in the digital world is also promising. The challenge is to attract those who need the knowledge and to help young users navigate the multitude of misinformation.

I anticipate and hope that this new take on fundamentally important questions will stimulate more fresh and informative research in the future. The well-being of our young people is at stake.

References

Brown, J. D., Steele, J. R., & Walsh-Childers, K. (Eds.). (2002). *Sexual teens, sexual media: Investigating media's influence on adolescent sexuality*. Lawrence Erlbaum Associates Publishers.

Brown, J. D., L'Engle, K. L., Pardun, C. J., Guo, G., Kenneavy, K., & Jackson, C. (2006). Sexy media matter: Exposure to sexual content in music, movies, television, and magazines predicts Black and White adolescents' sexual behavior. *Pediatrics, 117*(4), 1018–1027. https://doi.org/10.1542/peds.2005-1406

Chandra, A., Martino, S. C., Collins, R. L., Elliott, M. N., Berry, S. H., Kanouse, D. E., & Miu, A. (2008). Does watching sex on television predict teen pregnancy? Findings from a National Longitudinal Survey of Youth. *Pediatrics, 122*(5), 1047–1054. https://doi.org/10.1542/peds.2007-3066.

Greenberg, B. S., Brown, J. D., & Buerkel-Rothfuss, N. L. (Eds.). (1993). *Media, sex and the adolescent.* Hampton Press.

Healey, J. (2024, February 26). Beverly Hills middle school rocked by AI-generated nude images of students. *Los Angeles Times.* https://www.latimes.com/california/story/2024-02-26/beverly-hills-middle-school-is-the-latest-to-be-rocked-by-deepfake-scandal

Janfaza, R. (2023, July 17). Birth control will finally be sold over the counter. These youth activists pushed to make it happen. *Elle.* https://www.elle.com/culture/career- politics/a44555162/fda-approves-otc-birth-control-pills-explained/

Orenstein, P. (2024, April 12). The troubling trend in teenage sex. *The New York Times.* https://www.nytimes.com/2024/04/12/opinion/choking-teen-sex-brain-damage.html

ACKNOWLEDGMENTS

Most books, even those that are academic in nature, have origin stories. The idea for a book can often be traced back to a conversation, a news headline, or any number of observations that sparked the original idea. The origin of this book can be traced to an academic conference panel, held more than five years ago, in which scholars from across the country, including the editors of this book, met to discuss the challenges involved with collecting data from adolescents. At the time, we noted that most of the panelists were connected to Dr. Jane D. Brown. Each of us, for example, was Jane's doctoral advisee: Stacey graduated in 2005, Rebecca in 2012, and Jessica in 2013. We had all known each other previously, and we took time that day to share our favorite Jane stories, some of which were about her gifted approach to research and all of which were about her incredible kindness.

Fast forward two years ago. We recognized that Jane's work in *Sexual Teens, Sexual Media*, which we three had devoured, highlighted, and annotated as we embarked on our graduate studies, had not yet been updated. It seemed like a good idea, then, to undertake the task in hopes that we could continue Jane's work.

Given this, we must first acknowledge that who we are as researchers (and, one could argue, as feminists, mentors, and friends) is, in part, due to Jane's phenomenal mentorship, kindness, and investment.

There are others who have contributed significantly to this book. We thank all the authors who contributed chapters. We thoroughly enjoyed working with each group, and we are proud of the research that is included in this edited volume.

We want to thank Dr. Leticia Couto, now an assistant professor at DePaul University, who served as an editorial assistant and author. Her unwavering support throughout the entire process was appreciated. We were also fortunate to have a number of other graduate students who assisted us with conducting interviews, coding data, and organizing elements of this book: Christina Nickerson, Ron Price, Bailey Maykovich, and Jennifer Wybieracki. We appreciate their hard work. Stacey and Jessica would also like to thank Bruce Pinkleton, Dean of the Edward R. Murrow College of Communication, for his continued support of our research.

Stacey J.T. Hust: I'd like to thank Jessica and Rebecca, who helped make editing a book inspiring and fun. I could not have asked for two better collaborators. Many thanks to my dad, mom, and sister, who have always pushed me "to go out and do good." I must acknowledge Joshua M. Hust whose continued dedication and support have helped me realize several of my professional goals. Finally, to my daughters, thank you for inspiring me to ask the hard questions, and thank you for continuing to learn about this world with me.

Jessica Fitts Willoughby: I would also like to thank Rebecca and Stacey, who made the many hours we put into this book not only productive and rewarding, but enjoyable. Thanks to my parents, who always answered questions openly and honestly. Thanks to Shawn Willoughby for his continued support in all endeavors. And thank you to my children – you have helped me learn and grow in so many unexpected and wonderful ways.

Rebecca Ortiz: When Jessica and Stacey approached me to join them to edit this book, I did not hesitate for even a moment to say yes. As I anticipated, it has been an absolute pleasure working with them, as we care equally about doing high-caliber work that benefits young people, so thanks to them both. I would also like to thank my friends and family, especially my parents, who have always been my biggest fans. And thank you to all the young people in my life who have shared their thoughts and experiences with me so that I can continue to learn from you.

In closing, we thank the many young people who participated in our and others' research so that this volume could be curated. May some of you be inspired to join us on this journey.

INTRODUCTION

1

STATE OF THE FIELD

A Look at the Research Landscape on Teens, Sex, and Media

Jessica Fitts Willoughby, Stacey J.T. Hust, Rebecca Ortiz, and Leticia Couto

Teens today are immersed in media, with more control and choice over their media consumption than ever before. Research reveals that how and with which media teens engage can influence how they understand, make sense of, and behave in relation to their sexuality and sexual health (e.g., Coyne et al., 2019; Hust & Rodgers, 2018; Mori et al., 2019). In 2002, the seminal text *Sexual Teens, Sexual Media: Investigating Media's Influence on Adolescent Sexuality*, edited by Jane D. Brown, Jeanne R. Steele, and Kim Walsh-Childers, investigated the influence of media on adolescent sexuality. Its chapters covered everything from romantic portrayals in movies to sexual music lyrics. The authors used content analyses, surveys, and focus groups to study the sexual media landscape and its influence on adolescents.

The teens generally described in *Sexual Teens, Sexual Media* are now a generation of adults, some who may have become parents and now watch as their own teenage children navigate the increasingly complex mediated environment around them. Since those chapters were written, much work has been conducted in this area (e.g., Coyne et al., 2019; Mori et al., 2022). Meta-analyses have aggregated findings over multiple studies. One meta-analysis that looked at 59 studies, involving more than 48,000 participants, found that exposure to nonexplicit sexual media had a small but significant effect on sexual attitudes and behaviors, with media having a greater effect on adolescents than emerging adults, on boys than girls, and on White participants than Black participants (Coyne et al., 2019). This highlights how the impact of media may differ for individuals while still

DOI: 10.4324/9781032648880-2

broadly having an impact. However, the ways in which teens engage with media continue to constantly evolve.

For example, in 2002 when *Sexual Teens, Sexual Media* was published, original mainstream social media like MySpace and Facebook did not exist (appearing in 2003 and 2004, respectively). Now, contemporary social media, such as Instagram, YouTube, and TikTok, are ubiquitous in teens' lives. The internet and social media platforms are prominently used by adolescents in almost every part of the world, with young people living in poverty also often using mobile phones and social media (UNICEF, 2020). For example, 13- to 18-year-olds in the United States spend an average of nine hours a day with entertainment media, not including time spent using media for school or homework (Rideout & Robb, 2019). Among 16- to 29-year-olds in the European Union, 96% report using the internet daily, with 84% of them using it to access social media (Eurostat, 2023). Sub-Saharan Africa is one of the areas with the lowest percentage of people reporting access to the internet, but access has increased in recent years (Rheault & Reinhart, 2022). In South Africa specifically, internet access grew from 52% of people in 2019 to 66% in 2021, and adolescents and young adults in South Africa had greater access than older individuals, with 76% of 15- to 20-year-olds reporting access to the internet as of 2021.

In addition to changes in media access, there have been dramatic shifts in how teens consume content. With the advent of personal digital devices, teens can view media content on their own instead of co-viewing, in which multiple people view a program at the same time. In the United States, teens typically receive their first cell phone around 12 years of age (Richter et al., 2022), with 95% of 13- to 17-year-olds having access to one (Pew Research Center, 2018). In a study of nine- to 16-year-olds conducted across seven European countries and Japan, ten years old was the most common age at which a child first owned a mobile device, with children being more likely to get a phone a few years later in some countries (GSMA, 2015). For example, 37% of teens in Belgium who were surveyed said they first owned a phone at 12, which is often an age when youth enter a stage of schooling categorized by greater independence (e.g., junior high school) (GSMA, 2015). Access is not as ubiquitous in other locations, however. A study of nearly 5,000 10- to 15-year-olds from public schools in sub-Saharan Africa found that cell phone ownership rates were between 3% in Tanzania and 40% in Burkina Faso and South Africa (Wang et al., 2022).

Increased access to media content via private devices may mean that important discussions about the content to which teens are exposed do not occur between teens and their parents. Discussions with parents or other trusted adults about sexual-related media content can positively influence teens' interpretations of such content (e.g., Collins et al., 2003). In a novel study published in 2003, Collins and colleagues conducted a survey of 506 U.S. adolescents (ages 12–17) shortly after the popular television program *Friends* aired an episode in which a main character, Rachel, shared with another main character, Ross, that she was pregnant. In the episode, the characters repeatedly discuss the efficacy of condoms and describe the pregnancy as a result of a condom failure. The researchers found in their nationwide sample of adolescent *Friends* viewers that more than a quarter had seen the episode, and of those, 65% recalled the description of condom failure resulting in pregnancy. However, 40% of the adolescent viewers watched the episode with an adult, and 10% of those who watched the show discussed condom efficacy, or the effectiveness of condoms, because of the show. Adolescents who reported talking with an adult were more likely to report learning about condoms from the episode and had less reduction in condom efficacy beliefs. The authors concluded that media could serve as a healthy sex educator when media is used in conjunction with parental discussion.

Since that study, research has continued to emphasize the potential role of parents and discussions about media content as related to sexual behaviors. For example, in a meta-analysis that looked at the role of parental mediation on media effects related to sexual behavior, researchers found that active mediation (i.e., the process of discussing media content and encouraging the critical processing of such content) was related to reduced negative sexual outcomes among adolescents (Collier et al., 2016). The researchers also found small but significant effects on sexual health outcomes by restricting media and co-viewing media with youth (Collier et al., 2016). The authors concluded that parents may be able to mitigate some of the negative effects of media with mediation strategies, such as creating rules for media use and discussing the choices of characters and central themes, as well as engaging in media together. However, as teens are likely to own their own devices and may engage with media without parents around, such strategies may be difficult to implement.

Teens can also easily create and share content with others and view content on demand, which allows for increased personalization and control over their media diets, resulting in both positive and negative effects. For example, in a meta-analysis of 28 studies published since 2016 on sexting, which is the sending of sexual messages, photos, or videos via technology, among adolescents under the age of 18, approximately 19% have sent sexts (Mori et al., 2022). More than a third (35%) have received such messages, and 15% have forwarded sexts without consent from the original sender (Mori et al., 2022). Adolescents who engaged in sexting were more likely to have engaged in sexual activity, had multiple sexual partners, engaged in sex without using contraception, and experienced mental health concerns, including anxiety and depression (Mori et al., 2019). On the other hand, teens can also share and create content that expresses their opinions on controversial topics, giving them a voice and potentially spurring them to take action (see Willoughby et al., Chapter 19).

With all these changes in the types of media available and ways in which media are consumed by teens, we open this book with the results from a scoping review we conducted to examine the landscape of research about teens, sex, and media within the past ten years, at the time of writing (2013–2023). This review sought to answer questions, such as who conducts this research, what topics receive the most focus, and what adolescent populations are most often studied.

What we wanted to know and how we looked at it

We systematically collected literature across multiple research databases by searching for studies that focused on adolescents, media, and sexuality, using a combination of keywords representing relevant topic areas (e.g., teens, adolescents; romantic relationships, sex, sexuality; media, television, Instagram, video games, pornography). Based on our initial review, we created a list of the authors who conducted work in this area and then examined the publications listed on their Google Scholar profiles to see if they had other research we should include.

Adolescents/teens were generally defined as being between 13 and 21 years of age, but we also included articles that included participants up to age 29, as some studies spanned developmental stages (i.e., adolescence to emerging adulthood). However, we did not specifically look for studies that focused on participants in their late twenties (e.g., 24- to 29-year-olds). To be included, an article needed to include empirical research with a focus on adolescents and the topics of sex, sexuality, or relationships, and some form of media. Reviews and meta-analyses were excluded although were used to corroborate our literature search. Content analyses were only included if they focused on media content created by adolescents.

After completing the search, we additionally examined articles published between 2013 and 2023 in six journals that focus on the population or topic: *Journal of Children and Media*, *The Journal of Sex Research*, *Emerging Adulthood*, *Journal of Adolescent Health*, *Journal of Adolescent Research*, and *Youth & Adolescence*. Articles published in these journals that met the criteria were included in the review. Lastly, we used an artificial intelligence-powered research discovery tool (i.e., ResearchRabbit) to look at the articles we collected thus far to see if we missed other manuscripts related to our current selection. Once we had the complete dataset, we then reviewed the abstracts of all articles and removed articles that did not meet the inclusion criteria (primarily because the articles were not focused specifically on adolescents or were reviews). This resulted in a final sample of 210 articles.

Following collection of the sample, we downloaded meta-data extrapolated from the compiled articles including the title and journal. Then, we coded articles for several categories, such as the location of the work and the background of the authors, including their institutions and affiliations, as identified in the article. Additionally, we coded the gender of each article's lead author using either the pronouns used to describe the author in a biographical statement in the manuscript or on the scholar's personal or institutional webpage. If pronouns were not found, gender was not recorded for the scholar. We then coded the manuscripts by hand for manifest content, including the age range of the participants in the research and the nationality of participants in the research (i.e., U.S. or international sample). For latent content, which included the overall topic discussed in the article and the methods used, three coders coded the data, first establishing intercoder reliability with 12% of the sample randomly selected. Most of our categories had greater than 80% agreement among all coders, which is an acceptable level of agreement in terms of content analyses (Miles & Huberman, 1994). Some of our codes, particularly the ones more latent in nature, were lower than 80% but still above 70%. As scholars have noted previously, latent categories can be more challenging to code (e.g., Riffe et al., 2019), and so the 70% or higher intercoder reliability is appropriately rigorous.

What type of research is being conducted

The articles spanned 80 journals from multiple areas, including but not limited to, public health, medicine, communication, sexuality, and criminal justice. Multiple journals published more than ten articles on this topic: *Computers in Human Behavior (n = 20), Journal of Children and Media (n = 19), Journal of Adolescent Health (n = 13), Journal of Adolescence (n = 13), Journal of Interpersonal Violence (n = 10),* and *The Journal of Sex Research (n = 10).*

Among the topic areas that we coded, which included sexual health, sexual violence, romantic or sexual relationships, sexual identity, gender identity, and gender expression, a similar number of articles focused on sexual health, sexual violence, and relationships. A little more than a quarter (28.2%, *n* = 59) of the articles focused on sexual health, which included topics like contraception, sexually transmitted infection prevention and treatment, sex education, and sexual well-being. A little less than a quarter (23.4%, $n = 49$) focused on sexual violence, which included topics such as consent, coercion, and intimate partner violence, and 22% ($n = 46$) focused on relationships, which included topics such as romantic and sexual relationships and dating. Less prominent were articles that focused on sexual identity, gender identity, and gender expression (12.9%, $n = 27$). Although the study of the topic of gender identity and media has occurred for more than two decades now (e.g., Gauntlett, 2008), among the articles we collected from 2013 to 2023, more work focused on the topics of sexual health, sexual violence, and relationships. However, as articles could fit into multiple categories, it is also possible that sexual identity, gender identity, and gender expression were also often studied in conjunction with the other topics assessed.

Digital media communication channels (e.g., social media, text messaging) were more often a focus (89.0%, $n = 186$) than traditional media (e.g., television, movies) (18.7%, $n = 39$). Worth noting, sexting was a focus in 38.8% ($n = 81$) of the articles, and pornography in 12% ($n = 25$). Articles could fall into more than one of the categories mentioned above. These findings highlight the changes in the media landscape that have occurred over the last number of years, with research focusing primarily on digital media channels and a large proportion of work focusing on sexting. As noted by Mori et al. (2019), sexting has been an area of research since 2009 and the prevalence of sexting among youth appears to have plateaued (Mori et al., 2022). As digital media continues to be an area ripe for research and exploration, there is still a need for continued research among more traditional media outlets and understanding how, amid the changing media landscape, teens may engage with sexualized media in those contexts.

Research methods used

Researchers used a variety of methods, including surveys (71.3%, $n = 149$), focus groups (10%, $n = 21$), content analyses (9.1%, $n = 19$), interviews (8.1%, $n = 17$), mixed methods (7.2%, $n = 15$), experiments (5.7%, $n = 12$), and ethnography (1.4%, $n = 3$). Of those 149 studies that used survey research, only 19 (12.8%) were longitudinal. Our results highlight that the work conducted is most often quantitative and cross-sectional in nature, as evidenced by the prominence of survey research that is not longitudinal and the lack of experimental research. As research among scholars conducting this work also shows (see Ortiz et al., Chapter 2), there is a continued need for a mix of qualitative and quantitative methods to further our understanding of media and sex among adolescents. Researchers would bring great value to the research landscape by focusing on more robust designs that further our causal understanding of media on teen sexuality, as well as conducting more qualitative work that furthers our understanding of how teens make sense of the media and its potential impact. However, as researchers have noted, there are difficulties conducting this work (see Ortiz et al., Chapter 2), such that barriers and limited resources can make it difficult to reach these goals. Therefore, more resources should be invested to support scholars conducting highly impactful research in this field.

Who is the focus of this research?

The mean age of participants in our scoping review was 17.33 (SD = 3.49); however, only 127 of the articles reported mean ages. Some articles reported age ranges or years in school as a proxy for age. Participants' ages ranged from 12 to 29 years of age, although two studies had outliers who were greater than 29 years of age. Given some of the consent and access complexities associated with recruiting adolescents under the age of 18 (see Ortiz et al., Chapter 2), it is noteworthy that much of the research on these topics focused on participants under 18 years of age as this suggests many of these researchers could have experienced difficulties in recruiting, consenting, and assenting minors as part of the research process.

Nearly 60% of the articles had participants drawn only from the United States; 35.5% (n = 71) included participants from outside the United States; and 6% (n = 12) included both participants from the United States and outside the United States. For countries outside the United States, the most frequently represented countries were Belgium (n = 14, 6.7%), Australia (n = 9, 4.3%), the United Kingdom (n = 7, 3.4%), the Netherlands (n = 7, 3.4%), Italy (n = 6, 2.9%), Spain (n = 5, 2.4%), and Sweden (n = 4, 1.9%). Few studies had participants drawn from Asia (n = 4), Africa (n = 1), or South America (n = 2).

Who conducts research in this space?

Among the 210 articles assessed, 91.9% (n = 192) included a lead author from a higher education institution. Among those, 32.3% (n = 62) had a lead author in a communication-related college and department (e.g., College of Communication, Media Studies, Strategic Communication), 24.5% (n = 47) in public health or medicine colleges (e.g., College of Medicine, Nursing, Public Health, Kinesiology), 19.3% (n = 37) in psychology (e.g., Department of Psychology), and 4.2% (n = 8) from interdisciplinary units (e.g., Department of Psychology, Sociology and Politics). There were also publications from first authors in other units, including criminal justice, social work, and sociology, demonstrating how various fields contribute to the body of knowledge around adolescents, sex, and media.

More than 60% of the lead authors were women (63.6%, $n = 133$); 20.1% ($n = 42$) were men; 16.3% ($n = 34$) could not be identified by either the pronouns used in their biographies or on institutional webpages.

Most authors worked in teams, with only 3.3% ($n = 7$) of articles having a solo author. Some articles included up to 11 authors. The average number of authors was four. This highlights the team-based approach to conducting this work.

These findings highlight that researchers from a variety of fields are conducting this work in teams. Although we cannot directly assess from our compiled data if those teams were interdisciplinary, these findings highlight the potential for interdisciplinary work in the field. Previous research found that interdisciplinary work can be harder to publish and that people may be less productive, as evidenced by the number of journal articles; however, team-based work may have greater reach and impact (Leahey et al., 2017). Systems and processes that encourage interdisciplinary and collaborative research could benefit the field, such as leveraging existing large-scale survey data collection in other disciplines (e.g., public health) by including strong media measures and improving consideration of interdisciplinary work in the tenure process.

The trajectory of the field over time

Although not steady, there was an observable decline in the number of manuscripts published over the ten years (2013–2023) examined, with 31 manuscripts published in 2014 (highest) and ten manuscripts published in 2020 (lowest) (see Figure 1.1).

There may be several reasons for this decline, but we posit that this could be related to the difficulty in doing such work (see Ortiz et al., Chapter 2). Many of the topics in this field of research are controversial in certain countries. For example, the United States continues to experience controversy around the best ways in which to provide sex education content to teens (e.g., Schwartz, 2022) and around reproductive rights (Human Rights Watch, 2023). Coupled with universities that have suggested the removal of tenure or banned state funding for research that focuses on certain topics (i.e., sexuality, Mangan, 2023), conducting this work can present several challenges to researchers.

Historical events could also be influential in the amount of research conducted, either due to their relevance for study or due to their propensity to take time away from research in this specific topic area. The COVID-19 pandemic, for example, could have drawn researchers away from research

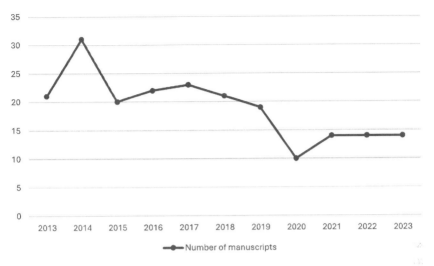

FIGURE 1.1 Publications in the field, 2013–2023.

in this field, either because of a transition in research focus to examine COVID-related communication phenomena or due to the fact that most researchers in this field of study are women and individuals from marginalized backgrounds (as discussed in Chapter 2) who are people who also experienced increased burdens during the COVID-19 pandemic and reduced research productivity (Douglas et al., 2022; Staniscuaski et al., 2021). However, the data indicate that the decline in articles was apparent even before 2020.

Directions for future research

We conducted a scoping review to provide context about the state of the field for research that focused on adolescents, sex, and media, but we also recognize that the review was not all-encompassing. Articles could have been missed in the search process or due to the specifics of our inclusion and exclusion criteria. For example, this review did not include a line of research on mobile interventions for sexual and reproductive health, including in international settings such as Africa (e.g., Olsen et al., 2018), that have documented success with scaling up interventions to reach additional populations (L'Engle et al., 2017). However, the exploration of the articles we included provides a strong understanding of the type of research being conducted in this space and provides direction for future research.

Based on this scoping review, we suggest researchers continue to aim to conduct rigorous research, whether it is longitudinal or experimental quantitative methods to determine the impact of media or more qualitative work to center teen voices about media impact. The fact that most quantitative work in this field used cross-sectional surveys leaves an avenue open for continued improvement. The team-based approach to research and the cross-disciplinary nature of those who engage in this work indicate the benefit of an interdisciplinary perspective. However, the controversial nature of some of the topics focused on and the additional resources needed to effectively conduct this work could lead to a decline in research in this area. Scholars must continue to work together to find ways to support rigorous research (e.g., through funding mechanisms and adequate time to conduct research with adolescents, which can take longer to shepherd through the IRB and/or community) and continue moving research in this area forward, especially given the increasing relevance of the topic today.

Additionally, the burden for advancing science in this area cannot fall solely on the researchers conducting work in this space. As noted, women are primarily the researchers publishing in this area, and external events, as evidenced by the COVID-19 pandemic, can negatively impact individual researcher's productivity. The field would benefit from increased structural support to advance researchers doing this work, and therefore the field in its entirety. Some possible suggestions include increased calls for collaborative research in which researchers share and build from data, increased structural resources, such as programs that provide modified duties, or reduced service loads during times in which researchers who conduct this work may be additionally burdened by "invisible" service (Oates, 2022), and increased resources that can allow for stronger samples and more robust methods of data collection to help support the science behind the findings.

References

Brown, J. D., Steele, J. R., & Walsh-Childers, K. (2002). *Sexual teens, sexual media: Investigating media's influence on adolescent sexuality*. Routledge.

Collier, K. M., Coyne, S. M., Rasmussen, E. E., Hawkins, A. J., Padilla-Walker, L. M., Erickson, S. E., & Memmott-Elison, M. K. (2016). Does parental mediation of media influence child outcomes? A meta-analysis on media time, aggression, substance use, and sexual behavior. *Developmental Psychology*, 52(5), 798–812. https://doi.org/10.1037/dev0000108

Collins, R. L., Elliott, M. N., Berry, S. H., Kanouse, D. E., & Hunter, S. B. (2003). Entertainment television as a healthy sex educator: The impact of condom-efficacy information in an episode of Friends. *Pediatrics*, 112(5), 1115–1121. https://doi.org/10.1542/peds.112.5.1115

Coyne, S. M., Ward, L. M., Kroff, S. L., Davis, E. J., Holmgren, H. G., Jensen, A. C., Erickson, S. E., & Essig, L. W. (2019). Contributions of mainstream sexual media exposure to sexual attitudes, perceived peer norms, and sexual behavior: A meta-analysis. *Journal of Adolescent Health*, 64(4), 430–436. https://doi.org/10.1016/j.jadohealth.2018.11.016

Douglas, H. M., Settles, I. H., Cech, E. A., Montgomery, G. M., Nadolsky, L. R., Hawkins, A. K., Ma, G., Davis, T. M., Elliott, K. C., & Cheruvelil, K. S. (2022). Disproportionate impacts of COVID-19 on marginalized and minoritized early-career academic scientists. *PLoS One*, 17(9), e0274278. https://doi.org/10.1371/journal.pone.0274278

Eurostat. (2023). *96% of young people in the EU uses the internet daily*. https://ec.europa.eu/eurostat/web/products-eurostat-news/w/ddn-20230714-1

Hust, S. J. T. & Rodgers, K. B. (2018). *Scripting adolescent romance: Adolescents talk about romantic relationships and media's sexual scripts*. Mediated Youth Series. Peter Lang Publishing.

Gauntlett, D. (2008). *Media, gender and identity: An introduction*. Routledge.

GSMA. (2015). *Children's use of mobile phones: A special report 2014*. https://www.gsma.com/solutions-and-impact/connectivity-for-good/public-policy/wp-content/uploads/2012/03/GSMA_Childrens_use_of_mobile_phones_2014.pdf

Human Rights Watch. (2023). *Human rights crisis: Abortion in the United States after Dobbs*. https://www.hrw.org/news/2023/04/18/human-rights-crisis-abortion-united-states-after-dobbs

L'Engle, K., Plourde, K. F., & Zan, T. (2017). Evidence-based adaptation and scale-up of a mobile phone health information service. *Mhealth*, 3, 11. https://doi.org/10.21037/mhealth.2017.02.06

Leahey, E., Beckman, C. M., & Stanko, T. L. (2017). Prominent but less productive: The impact of interdisciplinarity on scientists' research. *Administrative Science Quarterly*, 62(1), 105–139. https://doi.org/10.1177/0001839216665364

Mangan, K. (2023). *Indiana's funding ban for Kinsey Sex-Research Institute threatens academic freedom, IU president says*. https://www.hrw.org/news/2023/04/18/human-rights-crisis-abortion-united-states-after-dobbs

Miles, M. B., & Huberman, A. M. (1994). *Qualitative data analysis: An expanded sourcebook*. Sage.

Mori, C., Park, J., Temple, J. R., & Madigan, S. (2022). Are youth sexting rates still on the rise? A meta-analytic update. *Journal of Adolescent Health*, 70(4), 531–539. https://doi.org/10.1016/j.jadohealth.2021.10.026

Mori, C., Temple, J. R., Browne, D., & Madigan, S. (2019). Association of sexting with sexual behaviors and mental health among adolescents: A systematic review and meta-analysis. *JAMA Pediatrics*, 173(8), 770–779. https://doi.org/10.1001/jamapediatrics.2019.1658

Oates, M. (2022). *Invisible labor in academia*. https://www.academicdiversitysearch.com/invisible-labor-in-academia/

Olsen, P. S., Plourde, K. F., Lasway, C., & van Praag, E. (2018). Insights from a text messaging–based sexual and reproductive health information program in tanzania (m4rh): Retrospective analysis. *JMIR mHealth uHealth*, 6(11), e10190. https://doi.org/10.2196/10190

PEW Research Center. (2018). *Teens, social media & technology 2018*. https://www.pewresearch.org/internet/wp-content/uploads/sites/9/2018/05/PI_2018.05.31_TeensTech_FINAL.pdf

Rheault, M., & Reinhart, R. J. (2022). *Africa online: Internet access spreads during the pandemic*. https://news.gallup.com/poll/394811/africa-online-internet-access-spreads-during-pandemic.aspx#:~:text=Internet%20access%20in%20 Nigeria%2C%202019%20and%202021,to%2029%20(from%2030%%20 to%2047%%20access)

Richter, A., Adkins, V., & Selkie, E. (2022). Youth perspectives on the recommended age of mobile phone adoption: Survey study. *JMIR Pediatrics and Parenting*, 5(4), e40704. https://doi.org/10.2196/40704

Rideout, V., & Robb, M. B. (2019). *The common sense census: Media use by tweens and teens*. Common Sense Media Research. https://www.common sensemedia.org/sites/default/files/research/report/2019-census-8-to-18-full-report-updated.pdf

Riffe, D., Lacy, S., Fico, F., & Watson, B. (2019). *Analyzing media messages: Using quantitative content analysis in research*. Routledge.

Schwartz, S. (2022). *The sex ed battleground heats up (again). Here's what's actually in new standards*. https://www.edweek.org/teaching-learning/the-sex-ed-battleground-heats-up-again-heres-whats-actually-in-new-standards/2022/08

Staniscuaski, F., Kmetzsch, L., Soletti, R. C., Reichert, F., Zandonà, E., Ludwig, Z. M. C., Lima, E. F., Neumann, A., Schwartz, I. V. D., Mello-Carpes, P. B., Tamajusuku, A. S. K., Werneck, F. P., Ricachenevsky, F. K., Infanger, C., Seixas, A., Staats, C. C., & de Oliveira, L. (2021). Gender, race and parenthood impact academic productivity during the Covid-19 pandemic: From survey to action. *Frontiers in Psychology*, *12*. https://doi.org/10.3389/fpsyg.2021.663252

UNICEF. (2020). *Our lives online: Use of social media by children and adolescents in East Asia - opportunities, risks and harms*. https://www.unicef.org/indonesia/media/3106/file/Our-Lives-Online.pdf

Wang, D., Shinde, S., Drysdale, R., Vandormael, A., Tadesse, A. W., Sherfi, H., Tinkasimile, A., Mwanyika-Sando, M., Moshabela, M., Bärnighausen, T., Sharma, D., & Fawzi, W. W. (2022). Access to digital media and devices among adolescents in sub-Saharan Africa: A multicountry, school-based survey. *Maternal & Child Nutrition*, e13462. https://doi.org/10.1111/mcn.13462

2

THE MOTIVATIONS FOR AND CHALLENGES OF CONDUCTING RESEARCH WITH ADOLESCENTS ABOUT SEXUALITY AND MEDIA

Rebecca Ortiz, Jessica Fitts Willoughby, and Stacey J.T. Hust

In most parts of the world, adolescents under the age of 18 are minors/ children, a rightfully protected group of people to study, such that research conducted with youth undergoes stricter levels of ethical and legal scrutiny by review boards than research with adults (e.g., Office for Human Research Protections, 2016). Most research with adolescents will also require that both the youth participant assent and their parent or legal guardian consent to participation in a research study. Couple tasks like these with the topic of inquiry being sexuality, which is considered in many cultures a taboo topic, and you have an uphill battle for researchers studying adolescents, sexuality, and media.

Researchers also face significant and growing obstacles amid debates over sexual and reproductive healthcare access and evolving discourses on gender and sexual identities. Although international movements like #MeToo exposed the widespread nature of sexual misconduct and gender inequality (Mendes et al., 2018) and organizations like the International Lesbian, Gay, Bisexual, Trans, and Intersex Association, among others, provide advocacy for LGBTQ+ visibility and rights (Angelo & Bocci, 2021), political and social tensions around these and related issues remain. Look in almost every corner of the world and you will find examples of governments and interest groups engaged in dedicated efforts to limit access to sexual and reproductive healthcare, such as abortion and contraception, and undermine legal protections for LGBTQ+ people.

Examples are numerous, but here are three at the time of writing. In 2021, Hungary's government banned the dissemination of content deemed to promote homosexuality and gender-affirming healthcare to minors, a

DOI: 10.4324/9781032648880-3

move that is argued to marginalize LGBTQ youth by restricting representation in education and media and fueling discrimination and stigmatization (Beauchamp, 2021). In 2022, the U.S. Supreme Court overturned *Roe v. Wade*, eliminating federal protections for abortion access and leading several states to impose near-total bans on abortion with rare exceptions and limited time frames (Cohen et al., 2023; Guttmacher, 2024), deepening existing racial and gender inequities in the United States (Fuentes, 2023). In 2023, the Parliament of Uganda enacted the "Anti-Homosexuality Act," which prohibits any form of and promotion or recognition of sexual relations between people of the same sex, with a penalty of life imprisonment for committing "the offence of homosexuality" (UPPC, 2023). This Act, which was upheld by Uganda's Constitutional Court in 2024, has reportedly resulted in hundreds of arrests, tortures, and house evictions in the months following enactment (Reuters, 2024).

The urgency and complexity of these topics make conducting research in this area difficult, but critical. Experiencing challenges can lead researchers to significantly change the scope of their projects, potentially weakening their research, or even abandoning a project if the barriers appear insurmountable. When soliciting chapter contributions for this book, for example, we heard from researchers who were concerned about potential backlash to their research given recent legal restrictions in their geographic regions. Having experienced a variety of challenges ourselves in doing this work, we wondered about the motivations and challenges of others, and what advice they may have.

To answer this question, in September and October 2023, we emailed approximately 250 researchers who published research about adolescents, media, and sexuality within the past ten years (up to 2023) and asked them via an online survey about their motivations and challenges. All procedures were approved by the researchers' university institutional review boards prior to data collection. We examined descriptive statistics from closed-ended questions and individually coded the qualitative responses provided to open-ended questions using a thematic analysis. This chapter is a summary of those results. Spoiler alert: Although the challenges are plentiful, the motivations are as well.

Who were the researchers we heard from?

We heard from a diverse group of 53 researchers from various parts of the world, although most were currently employed in the United States (69.8%) at higher education institutions (83%) in such departments or colleges as media and/or communication, psychology, public health, medicine, nursing, sociology, women's and/or gender studies, and education.

Most identified their gender identity as a woman (n = 34, 64.1%), with 16 identifying as a man, two as nonbinary, and one who preferred not to answer. Fifteen (28%) identified as a sexual minority, nine as a racial and/ or ethnic minority, and three as having a disability.

The researchers represented a wide range of research experience, although most had ten or less years of experience doing this type of research. Only 16 respondents (30.2%) said that they had also conducted this type of research more than ten years ago. Age ranges of adolescence studied varied slightly, but the most common were middle adolescence (14–17) (n = 46) and late adolescence (18–20) (n = 34). The media most studied were social media (n = 46), television or video content (n = 28), pornography (n = 22), and text or direct messaging (n = 21), and the most common research methodologies researchers reported using were surveys (n = 48) and interviews (n = 28).

What are the challenges in doing this research?

When embarking on a research project with adolescents about media and sexuality, after determining the study purpose and methodology, researchers will quickly come up against the challenge of feasibility. In other words, how will they get this research project done? They must consider such questions as: Where will I access and recruit participants? How will I protect my participants' privacy and well-being during and after data collection? These are not unusual questions for any researcher working with human subjects to ask, but they are further complicated when the population is minors/children and the topics are media and sexuality.

Before a research study with adolescents is conducted, there are several gatekeepers a researcher must successfully navigate through. Funders must agree to fund the research. The researcher's institutional review board (IRB) must approve of the study protocol. School officials and/or survey sampling companies (as relevant) must agree to allow researchers to recruit and disseminate study materials in their respective spaces. Then, parents or guardians must agree to allow their adolescent child to participate. All this before adolescents can decide if they want to participate in a study on topics that directly affect them.

It therefore did not surprise us that the most common stages of research where our researcher respondents said that they experienced major challenges were during participant recruitment (n = 32), IRB/ethics review (n = 27), and data collection (n = 24). We have also experienced challenges at these research stages and were eager to learn about our peers' experiences. In analyzing their open-ended responses about these challenges, we identified two main themes, both of which are challenges unique in doing this work, such that they go beyond the normal obstacles of conducting human subjects research. These included (1) barriers and limitations driven by gatekeeper fears and moral objections and (2) dismissiveness and personal attacks for conducting sexuality and media research with adolescents.

Barriers and limitations driven by gatekeeper fears and moral objections

One would be hard-pressed to find a researcher who does not agree that their research with adolescents should undergo rigorous ethical review and include participant protections, but unfortunately, some gatekeepers judge the research from a place of fear and create unnecessary barriers and limitations. As one researcher wrote:

> There are so many barriers to accessing the population. If you make it through IRB, then you've got to find participants. If you don't have funding, it's nearly impossible. To get schools or organization[s] to collaborate feels like winning the lottery. It's fatiguing and all the resistance causes me to lose confidence and steam.

Some gatekeepers simply fear that asking young people anything about their sexuality will result in negative outcomes. One researcher mentioned that multiple gatekeepers can object to such inquiries: "Parents, school administrators, and IRB board members (primarily the latter two) are afraid of iatrogenic effects of asking about sexuality topics in surveys." Another researcher pointed out such barriers can affect recruitment:

> Recruitment was the major challenge, with very limited responses to social media requests, so we turned to schools. Many schools were afraid of the topic and would not participate. Some schools were positive and provided gatekeeper access through counsellors. The ethics approval process was driven by adult fears and demanded a number of safeguards that were not really necessary and were not taken up by the adolescents who participated.

Some of the researchers said that they experienced challenges from gatekeepers who considered their research topic "objectionable" or "unacceptable" and required them to change their study protocol in such a way that it watered down the rigor or accuracy of the data collected. As noted by one researcher, "The main difficulties were in the ways we could ask the questions to the adolescents. Some of the measures were not strong as a result of needing to be less direct." Another respondent provided a similar response: "The questions you can ask are always limited. And since parents must consent first, sample size/representativeness is always an issue."

These issues of access can become amplified when researchers study populations who experience marginalization and stigmatization, such as LGBTQ+ adolescents. One researcher wrote:

> One of the significant challenges I encountered while conducting research with adolescents about media and sexuality was recruiting a diverse sample of LGBTQ teens. Ensuring representation from various backgrounds, genders, sexual orientations, and sociocultural contexts was essential to capture a comprehensive range of experiences. This challenge required extensive outreach efforts, building trust with participants, and addressing potential barriers to participation, such as stigma or concerns about privacy. It was a vital aspect of the research process to ensure that the findings truly reflected the diversity within the LGBTQ adolescent community and provided valuable insights into their experiences with media and sexuality.

As this researcher notes, the barriers to conducting such studies may affect the quality or generalizability of the data. Additionally, gathering high-quality data from these populations is time-consuming and costly, which can pose additional challenges to researchers in higher education institutions who are pursuing tenure and promotion or dependent on funding for their salaries.

Dismissiveness and personal attacks for studying adolescent sexuality and media

Even if a researcher makes it through these recruitment and data collection challenges, they may still experience verbal attacks, intimidation, or dismissiveness for their topic of inquiry. For example, one researcher mentioned being dismissed by colleagues and other researchers for their work:

> There has often been a general tone of dismissiveness around my research when I've shared it with others … I felt patronized, like "Oh, there's ___ doing their little media research" or "Oh, yeah, that's ___, they do sexuality work." Trying to publish my work outside of media or gender journals (i.e., in "mainstream" psychology journals) has been challenging; my work is most often rejected, though accompanied by platitudes around how media is in fact important to study.

Others mentioned receiving insinuations or direct verbal attacks for being considered "perverts" or "pedophiles" for studying adolescent sexuality. One researcher shared:

> There is often just a general attitude that you are a pervert for doing this kind of research, that it moves beyond research into a kind of judgement about grooming or that you get some kind of thrill out of this. That disgusts me.

Such stigmatization may deter junior scholars and graduate students interested in these topic areas because they worry such attacks will negatively influence their marketability or career trajectories. Others, not surprisingly, stop the pursuit of their investigations once they have faced such attacks.

Why does anyone do this research then?

Although these challenges may sound overwhelming, many researchers, like us, persist. In fact, many of our researcher respondents said that they were driven by the desire to correct or address the same sex-negative, fear-based, and/or inaccurate messaging that drove their challenges, motivations to which we can also relate. They specifically mentioned the importance of studying media given its ubiquity in the lives of adolescents and adolescence being an important developmental period for sexuality and sexual health. One researcher wrote:

> Media is everywhere for adolescents and their go-to source for information about sexuality. It's also how they communicate and connect with each other. So conducting research to better understand their motivations, expectations, attitudes about using media to obtain sexual health information or access to sexual health resources, and understanding the barriers and facilitators to finding medically accurate, non-stigmatizing, non-judgmental information, and the positive and negative outcomes for accessing media for sexual health info are important areas to design more culturally relevant and responsive sexual health interventions for youth.

Another researcher echoed this sentiment when they wrote:

> I believe it is impossible to understand how adolescents are making decisions around their sexual health and practices in particular areas like contraception and abortion, if we do not understand their interactions with media of various kinds, and not only how they integrate

media with their own knowledge obtained from other sources, but how they are making decisions on what is trustworthy and accurate.

Several researchers also noted that they came to this field of study because of their personal experiences as an adolescent and/or having an identity that is underrepresented in the media. For example, one researcher wrote:

> My motivation to study media use and LGBTQ identity in adolescents is deeply personal. As a gay teenager, I experienced firsthand how online platforms influenced my journey of self-discovery and connection with the LGBTQ community. These experiences ignited my interest in understanding the impact of mass media and social media on LGBTQ youth. Through my research, I aim to uncover how these platforms can either empower or harm adolescents, drawing from my own experiences to contribute to a more supportive environment for LGBTQ youth.

Another researcher provided a similar response: "My personal experiences as a (closeted) queer adolescent. I am interest[ed] to understand ways that marginalized individuals can engage with mainstream or popular media in ways that are advantageous to their sexual health and development."

Some also said that they would continue this line of research because it was an important area to study with much still left to discover. "I think it's a vital and ever-changing topic," one researcher wrote, "as society and media changes, so does the experience of adolescents with media and sexuality." Another researcher similarly wrote:

> I feel that this continues to be an important and exciting area of research. As new technologies develop and adolescents embrace and use technology in new ways, it is important to understand the role of media in sexual socialization. I believe that we can empower adolescents to use media to enhance their sexual health.

Like this researcher, many of our respondents referenced their interest in improving the lives of adolescents and noted that there is still a lot unknown about adolescents' romantic and sexual lives.

What advice is there for future or current researchers?

Keep up the good fight and involve youth

When researchers were asked what advice they would pass along to future researchers, a common theme was the importance of, and how to better involve, adolescents in the research and, unlike some of the gatekeepers, acknowledge adolescents' agency and wisdom. For example, one researcher wanted to ensure that youth are at the center of this work. The researcher wrote: "It's important to adopt a child right's perspective and an intersectional one. Kids are also super smart and with it and have great ideas on what they want to see going forward." Another noted: "I recommend learning more about the needs of youth and understanding how to support them before, during, and after the research. It's important to conduct research *with* youth, and not simply *on* youth."

It was also mentioned by several researchers that adolescents often want to be involved because these topics are of interest to them. For example, one researcher said:

> Whilst it is a sensitive area, young people do want to talk about sex and sexuality. It's important to create an environment where they feel comfortable and if possible, have young people involved in the research process to ensure the research is youth centered (e.g., student researcher in similar age conducting interviews, youth consultation on study instruments).

Involving adolescents in research is also important to ensure accuracy and relevancy, especially in the ever-changing media landscape. One researcher, for example, wrote:

> Media platforms and modalities are constantly evolving, so don't focus your research on a specific media modality, rather focus on an underlying research question, motivation or outcome. Make sure to co-develop your research questions and protocols with youth as co-researchers so you're not biased or blinkered by ageism or other factors.

Another researcher also said: "Bring youth researchers onto your research team – they have the most relevant experiences and insights for this kind of research."

Since access to adolescents is one of the major challenges in doing this research, respondents encouraged future researchers to understand the gatekeeping challenges so that they can manage them appropriately and not let it weaken the rigor of their research. As one researcher wrote:

> You often have to access youth through schools, and between IRBs and school boards and principals, it's often hard to get these topics on to an actual survey. Managing the expectations of authority figures in conducting this research is very difficult.

Another researcher noted, however, that if done well, you can make it work: "Be very patient. It's doable but takes a lot of 'legwork' to develop trust and set up the proper infrastructure."

Some of the recommendations for navigating these difficulties included developing partnerships by building interdisciplinary networks. As one researcher shared, "Networks are really important to ensuring access to teens and children. Having partnerships outside of academia is the best way to ensure this." A few researchers also specifically suggested working in interdisciplinary teams to assist with these partnerships and improve the integrity of the research, "Collaborate with researchers from various fields such as psychology, sociology, and media studies to gain a holistic understanding of the complex interactions between media and sexuality among adolescents."

Continue to focus on conducting good science

Researchers also encouraged others in the field to conduct solid research, with a focus on strong research designs that put participants first. As one researcher noted: "[Doing this type of research is] difficult, but difficulty should never get in the way of good science." We agree with this statement wholeheartedly. The rigor of the research and ethics should be paramount in conducting this research.

Our respondents had some specific and different suggestions regarding what rigorous research might look like, such as collecting longitudinal (i.e., over time) data and employing different and methodologically sound research methods. As another researcher wrote, "Focus on longitudinal assessments, use well-validated measures, and address recruitment/attrition biases." Another noted the importance of "thinking critically about how to more accurately measure media use, making sure the study design and measures are culturally- and age- relevant." Others advised sound science through different methods:

> We're still in the stage where we need to do a ton of qual work to understand how and why people generally interact with the media … because each generation of adolescents works so hard to differentiate itself from the previous one and because technology continues to change at a pretty good clip. So, keep in touch with the qual people and keep a close eye on your instruments, if you're a quant- your tools will fall out of date fast.

What's the takeaway? Where do we go from here?

When studying adolescents, understanding media and sexuality is crucial. This is especially true during turbulent times where we see increased restrictions on sexual and reproductive healthcare access and LGBTQ+ protections. But we do not want to sugarcoat it. This work is challenging and not for the faint of heart. Scholars face several obstacles that make it difficult to conduct and publish this important research. Although individuals who conduct this research often have thoughtful reasons for doing this work, motivation alone will not overcome existing barriers. In fact, several of our respondents wrote that they would not continue this line of research because of the barriers. For example, one researcher said that they left the field because

> it had been frustrating to find outlets for my work; outside of a few "niche" journals, it seems scholars broadly dismiss the importance of media as a socialization force in the lives of adolescents, which is truly mindboggling to me. Furthermore, many of my colleagues did not know how to have a conversation about sexuality without being crude or dismissive.

Another wrote:

> I've pulled back on research in this area. As a researcher in the United States, it is logistically difficult to conduct this type of research. There is a lot of fear and strong feelings surrounding adolescent sexuality, which makes it difficult to obtain funding, IRB approval, etc. and it is very challenging to obtain a large sample of U.S. adolescents to discuss sexual topics.

Researchers and adolescents would therefore benefit greatly if institutions and funders considered how they might make this research more possible, whether through greater funding mechanisms that support increased quality of methodological rigor or improved processes at the institutional review board level that allow for increased adolescent autonomy in the consenting process. For example, adolescents who are at high risk for marginalization (e.g., sexual minority youth) may not participate in sexual health research if they are required to get parental/guardian permission because of concerns about their parent/guardian's negative attitudes about sexuality (Cwinn et al., 2021; Nelson et al., 2019). Many of these adolescents are therefore underrepresented in important research studies when we do not take these barriers into consideration and develop strategies that balance high ethical standards with greater participation access (Smith & Schwartz, 2019).

In addition to reducing institutional barriers, it is also important to shift conversations about sexuality away from fear-based morality arguments, such that we as educators, policy makers, researchers, parents/guardians, and citizens of the world must acknowledge that adolescent sexuality and media's role in its development should not be taboo topics. We cannot adequately ensure the healthy development of our children by ignoring the importance of sexuality and media in their lives.

We must also acknowledge that discussion of and research on these topics should not be conflated with predatory behaviors. Although efforts to limit access to sexual content and sexual health information or restrict sexual behaviors are often made under the guise of protecting children (e.g., Yarrow et al., 2014), these efforts prioritize stigma and shame, which can instead leave young people more vulnerable. We should instead champion efforts like media literacy education and discussions and education about important topics like sexual agency, consent, and identity. Systematic research efforts on these topics, such as how adolescents learn about sexuality from the media, can help us make sense of the best practices for healthy development so that we keep improving these efforts.

Researchers who persevere amid the challenges outlined above can provide critical insights to inform policies, educational programs, and interventions to improve young people's lives. For us, these rewards far outweigh the barriers and challenges because the work is meaningful and essential. Researchers in our survey noted that positively impacting youth's daily lives was one of the primary benefits of their work. We hope that, whether you are a researcher already in this space or an aspiring researcher, you will not be deterred by these challenges but instead inspired to join us because, despite the difficulties, the future is promising. The resilience of young people, along with the dedication of researchers and advocates in this space, signals a hopeful path forward. To succeed, researchers must continue to find and support each other, involve youth in their efforts, and do the best science possible.

References

Angelo, P. J. & Bocci, D. (2021, January 29). The changing landscape of global LGBTQ+ rights. *Council on Foreign Relations.* https://www.cfr.org/article/changing-landscape-global-lgbtq-rights

Beauchamp, Z. (2021, June 28). How hatred of gay people became a key plank in Hungary's authoritarian turn. *Vox.* https://www.vox.com/22547228/hungary-orban-lgbt-law-pedophilia-authoritarian

Cohen, D. S., Donley, G., & Rebouche, R. (2023). The new abortion battleground. *Columbia Law Review, 123*(1), 1–100. https://columbialawreview.org/content/the-new-abortion-battleground/

Cwinn, E., Cadieux, C., & Crooks, C. V. (2021). Who are we missing? The impact of requiring parental or guardian consent on research with lesbian, gay, bisexual, trans, two-spirit, queer/questioning youth. *Journal of Adolescent Health, 68*(6), 1204–1206. https://doi.org/10.1016/j.jadohealth.2020.07.037

Fuentes, L. (2023). Inequity in US abortion rights and access: The end of Roe is deepening existing divides. *Guttmacher Institute.* https://www.guttmacher.org/2023/01/inequity-us-abortion-rights-and-access-end-roe-deepening-existing-divides

Guttmacher Institute. (2024, May 2). *State bans on abortion throughout pregnancy.* https://www.guttmacher.org/state-policy/explore/state-policies-abortion-bans

Mendes, K., Ringrose, J., & Keller, J. (2018). #MeToo and the promise and pitfalls of challenging rape culture through digital feminist activism. *European Journal of Women's Studies, 25*(2), 236–246. https://doi.org/10.1177/1350506818765318

Nelson, K. M., Carey, M. P., & Fisher, C. B. (2019). Is guardian permission a barrier to online sexual health research among adolescent males interested in sex with males? *Journal of Sex Research, 56*(4–5), 593–603. https://doi.org/10.1080/00224499.2018.1481920

Office for Human Research Protections. (2016, March 18). Children: Information on special protections for children as research subjects. *HHS.gov.* https://www.hhs.gov/ohrp/regulations-and-policy/guidance/special-protections-for-children/index.html

Reuters. (2024, June 3). *Rights violations for Uganda's LGBTQ community escalating – pressure group.* https://www.reuters.com/world/africa/rights-violations-ugandas-lgbtq-community-escalating-pressure-group-2024-06-03/

Smith, A. U., & Schwartz, S. J. (2019). Waivers of parental consent for sexual minority youth. *Accountability in Research, 26*(6), 379–390. https://doi.org/10.1080/08989621.2019.1632200

UPPC. (2023, May 30). The Anti-Homosexuality Act, 2023, Acts Supplement. *The Uganda Gazette No. 36, Volume CXVI.* https://ulii.org/akn/ug/act/2023/6/eng@2023-05-30/source.pdf

Yarrow, E., Anderson, K., Apland, K., & Watson, K. (2014). Can a restrictive law serve a protective purpose? The impact of age-restrictive laws on young people's access to sexual and reproductive health services. *Reproductive Health Matters, 22*(44), 148–156. https://doi.org/10.1016/s0968-8080(14)44809-2

SECTION 1

Let's Talk About Mediated Sex

Using Media for Sexual Identity Development

3

SECTION 1 INTRODUCTION

Let's Talk About Mediated Sex: Using Media for Sexual Identity Development

Rebecca Ortiz

Adolescence is a critical time for sexual identity development. Starting around the ages of 10–13, young people go through significant physical, emotional, and behavioral shifts that extend into their late teens and early twenties (Sawyer et al., 2018). Although sexual development begins in infancy, it is this adolescent period of about ages 10–19 where sexual curiosity squarely meets social learning, such that peers and media play an ever-increasing influence on a young person's understanding of their identities and desires (e.g., Brown et al., 2005). Teens look to and compare themselves to others, in person and in the media, to make sense of who they are, such as how they should (or should not) express their gender and sexuality to meet socially desirable and culturally acceptable standards (Mazzarella, 2013).

Mainstream cultural norms around gender and sexuality are often based upon a cisgender heteronormativity, such that the standard is a binary gender of female or male that corresponds with the sex assigned at birth (i.e., cisgender) and sexuality operates between people of these two genders (i.e., heterosexual) (e.g., Pollitt et al., 2021). However, people's lived experiences demonstrate that these standards are limiting, especially for those who fall outside mainstream gender and sexuality norms and expectations (e.g., Gough et al., 2019; Tolman et al., 2016). Although more people, especially young people, are actively claiming their identities outside the cisgender binary (e.g., transgender, nonbinary, genderqueer) and heteronormativity (e.g., lesbian, gay, bisexual, pansexual) (e.g., Jones, 2024), identifying or expressing oneself outside of these standards carries risk, including social isolation and violence (see Ortiz et al., Chapter 2 for examples).

DOI: 10.4324/9781032648880-5

Media play a powerful role in challenging and disrupting these norms, allowing for more nuanced and authentic understandings of gender and sexuality. Although causation is hard to pin down, there is growing evidence that the increase in sexual and gender diverse media representations is associated with greater public support for lesbian, gay, bisexual, transgender, queer, and other non-straight or non-cisgender identities (LGBTQ+) rights and visibility (e.g., Zerebecki et al., 2021). The more we see diverse identities represented and normalized, the more accepting we are of their existence and rights. The next four chapters will explore some of the ways in which teens use media to develop and understand their gender and sexual identities amid this landscape of evolving cultural standards.

In Chapter 4, Hust and her team present findings from their interviews with teens from around the globe on how they interpret others' gender identities and sexual orientations based upon the person's media presentation. As mentioned by the researchers in this chapter, media play an important role in the social construction of gender and sexual orientation through culturally reinforcing and challenging portrayals and interactions. Since social media is popular among teens, two social media influencers who express their gender beyond traditional binary and heteronormative standards were presented to the teens, who were then asked to discuss how they determine the person's gender identity and sexual orientation. The teens also reported their level of agreement with aspects of the heterosexual script, and the researchers compared those responses to the teens' judgment of the social media influencers.

Chapter 5 presents a study by L'Pree Corsbie-Massay about how a cohort of first-year college students majoring in communication (therefore potential future media producers and content creators) made sense of media representations of sexuality in their favorite media content. The researcher challenged the students to critically analyze their favorite media content for presence or absence of sexuality and then explain how they came to those conclusions. The students' responses provide a nuanced and novel perspective on how young people subjectively navigate a media landscape where diverse media representations of sexuality are becoming more frequent, but heterosexuality remains normative and centered.

In Chapter 6, Mares and Chen discuss their study about how sexual and gender diverse youth (LGBTQ) may use media to facilitate conversations with their parents or identify their support about their sexual orientation and/or gender identity. As noted by the researchers, parental support is a strong predictor of positive mental health for LGBTQ youth, and while these teens want to talk with their parents about sex, the depth of the conversations is often lacking. Media depictions provide a way to open and facilitate conversations about these topics. The teens in this study were asked to provide an example of a media depiction that featured a person of their identity that they viewed with their parents and then report on how the experience went, positive or negative.

In Chapter 7, Dajches and co-authors explore how idolization of celebrities may play a role in the sexual self-concept of adolescent girls. The researchers note that teen girls sometimes develop parasocial relationships with their favorite celebs and use them as exemplars for developing their ideal romantic and sexual interactions, which the authors argue could influence how the girls perceive themselves as sexual beings. As noted by the researchers, past research on celebrity idolization has primarily focused on heterosexual teen girls, so they took extra effort to ensure that at least half of the girls in their study identified with a sexual identity other than straight/heterosexual (e.g., lesbian, bisexual). Doing so provided a unique opportunity to examine the association between celebrity idolization and sexual self-concept among a diverse group of adolescent girls and explore whether their sexual identity was an influential factor.

Together, these four chapters provide a glimpse into some of the work being done by researchers to better understand the importance and impact of media in the lives of young people as they develop and explore their gender and sexual identities.

References

Brown, J. D., Halpern, C. T., & L'Engle, K. L. (2005). Mass media as a sexual super peer for early maturing girls. *Journal of Adolescent Health*, *36*(5), 420–427. https://doi.org/10.1016/j.jadohealth.2004.06.003

Gough, B., Milnes, K., & Turner-Moore, R. (2019). Young masculinities across five European countries: Performing under pressure. *Journal of Youth Studies*, *24*(1), 77–90. https://doi.org/10.1080/13676261.2019.1695763

Jones, J. M. (2024, March 13). LGBTQ+ identification in U.S. now at 7.6%. *Gallup*. https://news.gallup.com/poll/611864/lgbtq-identification.aspx

Mazzarella, S. R. (2013). Media and gender identities: Learning and performing femininity and masculinity. In D. Lemish (Ed.), *The Routledge International Handbook of Children, Adolescents and Media* (pp. 305–312). Routledge.

Pollitt, A. M., Mernitz, S. E., Russell, S. T., Curran, M. A., & Toomey, R. B. (2021). Heteronormativity in the lives of lesbian, gay, bisexual, and queer young people. *Journal of Homosexuality*, *68*(3), 522–544. https://doi.org/10.1080/00918369.2019.1656032

Sawyer, S. M., Azzopardi, P. S., Wickremarathne, D., & Patton, G. C. (2018). The age of adolescence. *The Lancet Child & Adolescent Health*, *2*(3), 223–228. https://doi.org/10.1016/s2352-4642(18)30022-1

Tolman, D. L., Davis, B. R., & Bowman, C. P. (2016). "That's just how it is": A gendered analysis of masculinity and femininity ideologies in adolescent girls' and boys' heterosexual relationships. *Journal of Adolescent Research, 31*(1), 3–31. https://doi.org/10.1177/0743558415587325

Zerebecki, B. G., Opree, S. J., Hofhuis, J., & Janssen, S. (2021). Can TV shows promote acceptance of sexual and ethnic minorities? A literature review of television effects on diversity attitudes. *Sociology Compass, 15*(8), E12906. https://doi.org/10.1111/soc4.12906

4

MEDIATED IDENTITIES

A Qualitative Exploration of How Adolescents from Six Countries Make Sense of Gender Identity and Sexual Orientation in Media

Stacey J.T. Hust, Jessica Fitts Willoughby, Christina Griselda Nickerson, Ron Price, Rebecca Ortiz, Arian Karimitar, Joy Wanja Muraya, Hyelim Lee, Yoon-Joo Lee, and C. J. Janssen

More than half of the people in the world use social media at least once a month, and that number is projected to grow (Dixon, 2024). Usage is driven, in part, by adolescents and emerging adults (Auxier & Anderson, 2021), who may use these online spaces to explore and try on identities, including gender identity (Subrahmanyam & Šmahel, 2011). Rather than an unchanging absolute, gender is socially constructed through actively engaging with cultural and psychological dimensions in society. Unlike biological sex assigned at birth, gender is a phenomenon that is routinely performed and expressed through behavior, interactions with others, and one's own perceptions (West & Zimmerman, 1987).

A growing number of young people report having gender identities that differ from their birth-assigned sex or from social and cultural gender norms, including those who identify as transgender, nonbinary, or gender fluid (Diamond, 2020). Nonbinary and gender-fluid youth may identify as both male and female or neither male nor female (Diamond, 2020). In this chapter, we defined gender identity and sexual orientation in alignment with the glossary of terms provided by the Gay & Lesbian Alliance Against Defamation (GLAAD, 2024). Gender identity is a person's self-identified gender and internal sense of self, which is not outwardly visible to others (unlike gender expression), and which may or may not align with a person's sex at birth. Gender identity and sexual orientation are distinct aspects of a person's identity, and their meanings can vary across different cultures. Sexual orientation describes a person's physical, romantic, and/or

DOI: 10.4324/9781032648880-6

emotional attraction to others, which may or may not be based upon a person's and other's gender identity and/or expression.

Overall, media play an important role in the social construction of gender and beliefs about sexual orientation through on-screen portrayals and social media interactions (e.g., West & Zimmerman, 1987). Social media has provided an outlet for non-celebrities, including teens, to gain global stardom (Brooks et al., 2021). Social media influencers (SMIs) are individuals who have a significant number of relationships and followers on social media and can influence others through content production, distribution, interaction, and personal appearances on the internet (Enke & Borchers, 2021). Corporations around the world rely on SMIs. For example, influencer marketing constitutes 60–70 percent of online retailer Jumia Nigeria's marketing efforts (Fakeye & Ayoola, 2023). Similarly, qualitative research with teens in the Middle East pointed out that SMIs play an indirect role in how Egyptian youth construct and negotiate their online identities (Ezzat, 2020).

SMIs can reinforce or challenge gender-conforming portrayals (e.g., Parkins & Parkins, 2021). Some gay male beauty influencers, for example, engage in a production of femininity that was previously reserved for female beauty influencers but for which they receive recognition and support based on their appearance of authenticity and individuality (Chen & Kanai, 2022). With such diverse content, adolescents can follow accounts of people whose gender identity or sexual orientation they relate to or whose identities differ from their own. Furthermore, adolescents may try to mimic established SMIs to increase their own social media reach (Caro-Castaño, 2022). Such gendered interactions then become internalized and can affect beliefs in gender roles, such as beliefs in heterosexual scripts (Seabrook et al., 2016) and perceptions of others' gender identities or sexual orientation (Smith & Smith, 2016). Given this, our study included interviews with teens to explore how they make sense of the gendered images they see on social media, specifically images of globally popular SMIs who challenge the perception that gender is binary.

Method

Given the global reach of social media, we wanted to explore how adolescents from across the globe make sense of gendered images of SMIs. We acknowledge these individuals live in different national contexts but are residents in a shared global social media environment. Therefore, we did not compare participants from different cultures but instead highlighted the importance of adopting a cross-cultural perspective when studying social media and adolescents. Furthermore, we relied on each participant's self-identified labels and meanings of gender identity and sexual orientation to understand how they make sense of their and others' identities; however, we used the labels (e.g., identities, pronouns) self-identified by the media stars (e.g., SMIs) when discussing them even if the participants did not agree with or accept the media stars' identities. Our goal was to allow for various individual understandings of gender identity and sexual orientation while also acknowledging that each person is the best judge of their identity.

Sample and procedure

We recruited 17 participants from Brazil, Iran, Kenya, Nigeria, South Korea, and the United States through direct contact and snowball sampling. Participants not from the United States were at least 18 years of age per Institutional Review Board approval. U.S. participants ranged in age from 15 to 20 years old (see Table 4.1 for relevant demographic information). Both English and Portuguese, the official languages of the United States and Brazil, respectively, include terms (e.g., use of pronouns) that can be used to describe nonbinary people. The U.S. and Brazilian governments provide their citizens with options to legally identify as nonbinary. The Iranian and South Korean governments acknowledge that individuals may identify as a gender different from the sex they were assigned at birth, but these individuals often face significant discrimination and violence (Cho & Richards, 2023; Human Dignity Trust, 2023). At the time of this writing, neither the government of Kenya nor Nigeria recognizes a gender beyond male or female (Human Dignity Trust, 2024; Nyangweso, 2007).

Prior to participating in an interview, participants provided consent (and if under 18, we first obtained parental consent before teens assented). Participants then completed a survey that asked about their media use, their favorite media star (e.g., celebrity or SMI), background demographics, and responses to the Heterosexual Script Scale (HSS). The HSS includes statements about stereotypical and gendered romantic and sexual interactions, such that heterosexual relationships are considered the norm, and women and men play complementary but unequal roles (Seabrook et al., 2016; see Measurement Appendix). All media-use surveys, aside from South Korea, were administered in English and tailored to ask participants about media popular in their country.

Trained interviewers facilitated 90- to 120-minute virtual conversations, conducted in the participants' native languages, on Zoom using a semi-structured interview protocol, which was piloted before data were formally collected. We asked participants to discuss the gender identity of their favorite media star, and we showed them two images of globally popular SMIs who do not conform to binary gender identities and identify as members of the LGBTQ+ community. The first photo was of a male beauty

TABLE 4.1 Participants' demographics and beliefs in the heterosexual script

Participant	Gender	Sexual orientation	Country	Age	Beliefs in the heterosexual script				Overall Mean	Heterosexual Script Adherence
					Courtship and commitment	Men as powerful initiators	Men value women's appearance	Sex defines masculinity; women set sexual limits		
Ola	Man	Heterosexual	Nigeria	19	4.00	4.75	5.00	2.40	4.00	Endorses HSS
Milad	Man	Heterosexual	Iran	20	3.50	4.00	3.00	3.00	3.36	Endorses HSS
Ravio	Man	Heterosexual	U.S.	15	2.88	3.00	4.00	2.80	3.14	Endorses HSS
Tina	Woman	Heterosexual	Kenya	20	1.63	4.50	2.60	4.80	3.09	Endorses HSS
Neda	Woman	Questioning	Iran	23	2.13	3.50	3.00	4.00	3.00	Endorses HSS
Sarah	Woman	Bisexual	U.S.	16	2.38	3.50	3.40	3.20	3.00	Endorses HSS
Ijun	Man	Heterosexual	S. Korea	23	2.50	2.50	3.80	2.40	2.77	Endorses HSS
Jian	Woman	Heterosexual	S. Korea	22	2.38	2.75	3.20	2.80	2.73	Endorses HSS
Essie	Woman	Questioning	Kenya	18	2.38	3.00	2.00	2.80	2.50	Neutral
Eyinju	Woman	Heterosexual	Nigeria	–	2.63	2.75	1.80	2.80	2.50	Neutral
Carlos	Man	Heterosexual	Brazil	18	1.38	3.50	3.00	2.40	2.36	Rejects HSS
Arthur	Man	Heterosexual	U.S.	15	2.38	2.75	2.20	2.20	2.36	Rejects HSS
Thais	Woman	Heterosexual	Brazil	18	1.75	2.75	2.00	2.40	2.14	Rejects HSS
Myah	Woman	Heterosexual	U.S.	17	1.88	2.75	2.00	1.80	2.05	Rejects HSS
Jenny	–	Bisexual	U.S.	16	1.38	2.25	3.20	1.20	1.91	Rejects HSS
Ang	Man	Heterosexual	U.S.	15	1.13	2.50	1.80	1.00	1.50	Rejects HSS
Lily	Woman	Bisexual	U.S.	15	1.50	1.50	1.00	1.00	1.27	Rejects HSS

Notes: Items were asked on a 1 to 5 strongly disagree (1) to strongly agree (5) scale.

vlogger who wore fashionable clothes, makeup, and jewelry. The second image was a profile photo of a nonbinary actor who had long curly hair and wore a blue plaid shirt. Participants were asked to discuss their impressions of these SMIs.

We used Zoom's recording and auto-transcription features to record and transcribe the interview data from English-language interviews, and for non-English interviews, recordings were securely submitted to an audio transcription and translation program (i.e., HappyScribe). Research team members who spoke the native language in which the interview was conducted verified the transcripts for accuracy. Three individuals, including the first author, analyzed the data in MAXQDA using a thematic analysis approach, and patterns in the data were identified (Braun & Clarke, 2006). The coding process was iterative, including multiple meetings in which coders shared results with the larger research team, which further informed coding efforts. Below, we report the main themes indicating how our participants made sense of gender identity in relation to their personal media experiences, the SMIs to which they viewed in the interview, and their level of agreement with stereotypical statements about heterosexual relationships (i.e., the HSS).

Youths' adherence to the heterosexual script

Youths' responses to the HSS items (a scale developed with a U.S. sample, Seabrook et al., 2016) indicated some youth endorsed traditional heterosexual scripts, while others rejected them. Youth who disagreed with traditional heterosexual scripts included men and women who lived either in the United States or Brazil. Youth who endorsed traditional heterosexual scripts included a diverse group of men and women living in Iran, Kenya, Nigeria, the United States, and South Korea. Within our sample, a participant's sexual orientation was not associated with the rejection of heterosexual scripts as some participants who identified as bisexual or questioning reported endorsing these traditional beliefs (i.e., Neda & Sarah), while others with these identities rejected them (i.e., Jenny & Lily). See Table 4.1.

Making sense of gender identity

Regardless of their endorsement of heterosexual scripts, youth used traditional physical attributes, such as physical stature, hairstyle, and clothing, to describe and determine the gender identity of their favorite media stars and the SMIs they were shown. For example, Arthur, a heterosexual man from the United States, mentioned that Dwayne "The Rock" Johnson, a U.S. actor, was clearly a man because of his muscularity and athleticism.

Sarah, a bisexual woman from the United States, said that Billie Eilish, an American singer-songwriter, "uses the way she dresses to define her femininity." Milad, a heterosexual Iranian man, identified that his favorite musicians were men, and when asked how he knew these musicians were men, he said that "their gender is obvious."

Most participants identified the first SMI as a woman, even though the influencer was a male beauty vlogger who uses he/him pronouns. When Myah, a heterosexual U.S. woman, was identifying him as a woman, she said: "And it looks like they have like lipstick or something on, maybe a little bit of makeup." It is worth noting that Myah referred to the SMI as "they," even as she identified him as a woman. Similarly, Tina, a heterosexual Kenyan woman, and Ravio, a heterosexual man from the United States, said that the SMI's pose and makeup indicated that he was a woman. Neda, an Iranian woman questioning her sexuality, mentioned these same physical features as evidence that the influencer was not male, but she also considered whether the SMI was female, nonbinary, or transgender. Such openness about nonbinary gender may be unusual among Iranians, given that LGBTQI+ individuals in Iran are subject to violence and discrimination (The Iran Primer, 2024). In fact, Neda's response was very similar to Jenny's, who rejects heterosexual scripts. Jenny, who is questioning both her gender and sexuality, identified the first SMI as someone who "maybe presents in between nonbinary or female." After youth were informed the first SMI identified as a man who uses he/him pronouns, some explained their thinking. For example, once Carlos, a Brazilian heterosexual man, knew he misidentified the first SMI as a woman, he said:

> Actually, like just it's, I didn't expect that, but I can't make any conclusion like, because he's a man or a woman, you know, like it doesn't matter if you know, like that's not relevant, like he's a man or woman, to my conclusion about him.

The second image we showed participants was of a nonbinary SMI who wore makeup and had long, brown curly hair. Although youth had readily identified the gender of the first SMI, they seemed more hesitant to identify the gender identity of the second one. Both Sarah and Arthur questioned whether the second SMI was a woman or a man, because they seemed more aware that individuals may identify as a gender different than their outward gender expression. Sarah said: "Also looks feminine, or more like woman, or I don't know. Actually, I feel like, so both ways, like a nonbinary kind of situation, I'm not ... I'm not sure." Similarly, Jian, a heterosexual South Korean woman, seemed to struggle to identify the gender of the second SMI. "I may be biased," Jian said, "but she seems to have a more masculine appearance than feminine. It's like she's a woman transitioning to a man while wearing men's clothing."

In fact, some participants were hesitant to draw conclusions about the second SMI based on a photo alone, even though they had done so earlier in the interview when describing the first SMI. Essie, a Kenyan woman questioning her sexuality, said: "It's really hard to form an opinion based on just a photo." Lily, a bisexual woman from the United States, also noted that it would be hard to identify the second influencer's gender identity based on the photo but added that "in this photo" the influencer appears more feminine due to "the stereotypical things like the clothes, the hair, the makeup."

Some of the teens who adhered to more traditional gender roles struggled to reconcile their perceptions of the SMIs with information about how the individuals identified. Eyinju, a heterosexual Nigerian woman, said that she was confused by the photo of the second SMI, and she struggled to make sense of how the SMI could identify as nonbinary. "Well, she has breasts," Eyinju said. "That's the only thing I can see, but mainly for when you look at that you can tell that she's a woman." Similarly, Milad readily identified the second influencer as a woman and did not question this even as the interviewer explained that the influencer identifies as nonbinary. Jian was also confused by the second influencer's gender identity and went on to express discomfort with meeting nonbinary people in real life. Jian said: "I'm just a little reluctant about 'they' or 'them' … I don't understand. You are biologically male, but you think you are female. I don't really want to get too close to those people."

Although Jian was the only participant who acknowledged discomfort with nonbinary people during the interview, most agreed that individuals who are older than them, such as their parents or grandparents, would not be accepting of such an identity. Carlos said that older people would treat the second influencer differently if they knew that the SMI did not identify as a woman. Similarly, Sarah noted that older individuals grew up in a different era, which may explain why they would not understand nonbinary people. She perceived that nonbinary people are more common now than historically.

Conversely, two participants, both of whom identify as bisexual, said that older individuals would be accepting. Lily, who conducted her interview in front of a large pride flag that hung on the wall of her bedroom within her parents' home, was confident that her parents would accept either of the SMIs. Sarah said that older people would understand nonbinary people or those who identified as LGBT, because "there's a lot more LGBT artists coming out." These perspectives emphasize the subtle differences in opinions, indicating that the level of acceptance toward gender identities and sexual orientations can greatly alter depending on individual experiences and exposure.

Perceived association of gender identity with sexual orientation

Our participants regularly associated gender identity with sexual orientation. For example, many participants assumed that the SMIs were gay or lesbian once they knew the SMIs identified as nonbinary or rejected traditional gender norms. Sarah believed that the first SMI was gay because he did not conform to a traditional masculine identity. Tina also assumed that he was gay and specified that his sexuality would affect how he behaved in a relationship. Tina said: "I will say that he will look for a guy who is gay, but he would be, will be the lady like. Will be the girlfriend. Yeah." Myah also noted that she would make assumptions about sexual orientation based on someone's gender identity. She said:

> Well, I guess sometimes like, let's say, like a girl, might act like more masculine, like you might like assume that they're lesbian and like, same with guys like, if they act more feminine, you might assume that they're gay.

In addition, Thais's description of her favorite media star demonstrates the confusion that exists between gender identity and sexual orientation. Thais, a heterosexual Brazilian woman, identified her favorite media star as gay, but then she struggled to identify which pronoun to use. She explained: "I think it's like this, me speaking of him, I say 'him,' right? Like he's homosexual, right? ... Like, for me, at least, I mean him." Thus, Thais tried to reconcile the media star's gender identity with his sexual orientation.

Furthermore, when discussing the gender identity of their favorite media stars, youth often referred to the media star's previous relationships. Both Carlos and Arthur said that their favorite media stars identified as men because each celebrity had been in romantic and sexual relationships with women. Neda noted that Taylor Swift, an American singer-songwriter, is a heterosexual woman because she writes about relationships with men in her lyrics, and she also has dated men in real life. Many participants, however, struggled to make sense of media stars who portrayed characters displaying different gender norms or a different sexual orientation than the star does in real life. Arthur, for example, thought it was funny when Dwayne Johnson portrayed a less masculine male in *Jumanji II*, because, in his opinion, such a portrayal was incongruent with Johnson's real-life gender expression.

Although the presence of LGBTQ+ and nonbinary people has increased in the media (Gay & Lesbian Alliance Against Defamation Media Institute, 2023), our participants were still unclear on how to reconcile these identities. Jenny identified one possible explanation for such confusion. She said that the media she consumes often includes nonbinary characters, but she acknowledged that she did not know much about the sexual lives of nonbinary people. "Now I'm thinking about [it], like I do see nonbinary characters, but a lot of the time they don't have like a love interest," Jenny said. As Jenny acknowledges, the challenge of relying on on-screen depictions to make sense of real-life identities is that the viewer is dependent on the limited media portrayals of LGBTQ+ and nonbinary people.

Discussion

Teens think they are more open than previous generations, and in many ways, they are; yet these results indicate that participants still rely on traditional gender cues and biological sexual characteristics (e.g., when Eyinju identified an SMI as female because they had breasts) to identify individuals' gender identity. In many of our participants' countries, structural challenges, such as a lack of linguistic specificity and few laws supporting gender identification and sexual orientation, exist, which makes it challenging to discuss gender and sexual minorities. After struggling to accurately identify the gender identity of the first SMI, many of our participants were hesitant to try and identify the gender of the second SMI. Such findings suggest that the participants' first experience may have served to prime many individuals to the possibility that gender is not binary. Priming refers to the influence of media exposure on subsequent judgments of media or nonmedia content (Roskos-Ewoldsen et al., 2007). Additional experimental research should examine how younger generations may be primed in their perceptions of gender identities and sexual orientations.

Our results suggest that these participants often drew conclusions about gender identity based upon their perceptions and understanding of sexual orientation. Multiple participants said that their favorite media stars were either men or women, because they had witnessed them engage in heterosexual relationships. These participants' presumption is that an individual who is heterosexual will identify as either a man or a woman, which is not necessarily accurate. This misconception highlights the need for media portrayals to include diverse representation, and the importance of such content to make clearer distinctions between gender identity and sexual orientation.

Additionally, this is one of the first studies, to our knowledge, in which adolescents from around the world responded to the statements in the

Heterosexual Script Scale. Our sample is too small to generalize about the reliability of the scale with different populations, but our findings suggest that the scale may be applicable to youth outside of the United States. In general, the participants' quantitative responses to the HSS were consistent with their qualitative data, with some notable exceptions. For example, when considering the quantitative HSS responses of our participants, Neda was identified as one who endorsed such scripts, yet her qualitative interview suggested she rejects some gender norms. It is possible that among other Iranians, Neda's beliefs in heterosexual scripts (overall mean of 3.0 on a 5.0 scale) would be viewed as rejecting such beliefs. Future research should test the reliability of using the HSS with international populations to better understand how nationality and culture are associated with these beliefs.

Although our findings provide a unique glimpse into how adolescents living in countries across the world make sense of mediated gender identity and sexual orientation, this study has its limitations. Given the small sample from each nation, our findings are not generalizable, and our ability to make cross-cultural comparisons is limited. Despite this limitation, our findings suggest that it is important to consider a cross-cultural population when doing this work, and future qualitative research should look at learning how youth from other countries not represented here make sense of gender identity.

Conclusion

As West and Zimmerman (1987) noted, gender is socially constructed through interactions. Although adolescents expect that individuals their age will be more aware and accepting of nonbinary gender than older adults, our results indicate that these youth still relied on traditional gender cues and biological sex characteristics when trying to determine one's gender identity. In fact, our results illustrate how adolescents engage with and perceive others as "doing gender" while drawing from their experiences in identifying the gender identity of the first SMI, who did not adhere to traditional gender expression, to make sense of the second nonbinary SMI's gender identity. Teens were also more likely to decide that gender could not be determined by image presentation alone after being corrected about a given SMI's gender identity that differed from the outward presentations in his profile picture. This highlights how exposure to people of all types of gender identities and sexual orientation, including through mediated portrayals, can potentially impact teens.

References

Auxier, B., & Anderson, M. (2021). *Social media use in 2021*. Pew Research Center. https://www.pewresearch.org/internet/2021/04/07/social-media-use-in-2021/

Braun, V., & Clarke, V. (2006). Using thematic analysis in psychology. *Qualitative Research in Psychology, 3*(2), 77–101. https://doi.org/10.1191/1478088706qp063oa

Brooks, G., Drenten, J., & Piskorski, M. J. (2021). Influencer celebrification: How social media influencers acquire celebrity capital. *Journal of Advertising, 50*(5), 528–547. https://doi.org/10.1080/00913367.2021.1977737

Caro-Castaño, L. (2022). Playing to be influencers: A comparative study on Spanish and Colombian young people on Instagram. *Communication & Society, 35*(1), 81–99. https://doi.org/10.15581/003.35.1.81-99

Chen, S. X., & Kanai, A. (2022). Authenticity, uniqueness and talent: Gay male beauty influencers in post-queer, postfeminist Instagram beauty culture. *European Journal of Cultural Studies, 25*(1), 97–116. https://doi.org/10.1177/1367549421988966

Cho, H. E., & Richards, E. R. (2023). *Why South Korea can't pass anti-discrimination laws*. Asialink. https://asialink.unimelb.edu.au/insights/why-south-korea-cant-pass-anti-discrimination-laws

Diamond, L. M. (2020). Gender fluidity and nonbinary gender identities among children and adolescents. *Child Development Perspectives, 14*(2), 110–115. https://doi.org/10.1111/cdep.12366

Dixon, S. J. (2024). *Number of worldwide social network users from 2017 to 2028 (in billions)*. Statista. https://www.statista.com/statistics/278414/number-of-worldwide-social-network-users/

Enke, N., & Borchers, N. S. (2021). Social media influencers in strategic communication: A conceptual framework for strategic social media influencer communication. In *Social Media Influencers in Strategic Communication* (1st ed., pp. 7–23). Routledge.

Ezzat, H. (2020). Social media influencers and the online identity of Egyptian youth. *Catalan Journal of Communication & Cultural Studies, 12*(1), 119–133. https://doi.org/10.1386/cjcs_00017_1

Fakeye, O., & Ayoola, M. (2023). Social media influencers in retail marketing in Nigeria. *International Journal of Women in Technical Education and Employment, 4*(1), 85–95.

Gay & Lesbian Alliance Against Defamation Media Institute. (2023). *Where we are on TV*. Gay & Lesbian Alliance Against Defamation. https://assets.glaad.org/m/7c489f209e120a11/original/GLAAD-2023-24-Where-We-Are-on-TV.pdf

GLAAD. (2024). *GLAAD Media Reference Guide*. 11th ed. https://glaad.org/reference/#guide

Human Dignity Trust. (2023). *Iran*. Human Dignity Trust. https://www.humandignitytrust.org/country-profile/iran/

Human Dignity Trust. (2024). *Nigeria*. Human Dignity Trust. https://www.humandignitytrust.org/country-profile/nigeria/

Nyangweso, M. (2007). *Female circumcision: The interplay between religion, culture, and gender in Kenya*. Orbis Books.

Parkins, M., & Parkins, J. (2021). Gender representations in social media and formations of masculinity. *Journal of Student Research*, *10*(1). https://doi.org/10.47611/jsr.v10i1.1144

Roskos-Ewoldsen, D. R., Klinger, M. R., & Roskos-Ewoldsen, B. (2007). Media priming: A meta-analysis. *Mass media effects research: Advances through meta-analysis*, *50*, 53–80.

Seabrook, R. C., Ward, L. M., Reed, L., Manago, A., Giaccardi, S., & Lippman, J. R. (2016). Our scripted sexuality: The development and validation of a measure of the heterosexual script and its relation to television consumption. *Emerging Adulthood*, *4*(5), 338–355. https://doi.org/10.1177/2167696815623686

Smith, J. S., & Smith, K. E. (2016). What it means to do gender differently: Understanding identity, perceptions and accomplishments in a gendered world. *Humboldt Journal of Social Relations*, *38*, 62–78. https://doi.org/10.55671/0160-4341.1034

Subrahmanyam, K., & Šmahel, D. (2011). Constructing identity online: Identity exploration and self-presentation. In *Digital Youth: The Role of Media in Development* (pp. 59–80). Springer.

The Iran Primer. (2024, April 25). *U.S. Report: LGBTQI+ Persecution in Iran.* https://iranprimer.usip.org/blog/2024/apr/25/us-report-lgbtqi-persecution-iran#:~:text=Violence%20and%20Harassment:%20LGBTQI%20persons, for%20information%20on%20LGBTQI+%20persons.

West, C., & Zimmerman, D. H. (1987). Doing gender. *Gender and Society*, *1*(2), 125–151. https://doi.org/10.1177/0891243287001002002

5

MAKING SENSE OF MEDIATED SEXUALITY

Examining the Perceptions of First-Year College Students

Charisse L'Pree Corsbie-Massay

Audiences make sense of the world by engaging with media content. Adolescence can be characterized by a perceptive shift in awareness as young people become aware of how media informs interpretations of reality. This multifaceted inflection point includes changes in physical development, cognitive processing, and media engagement. Multiple content analyses have demonstrated that representations of (hetero)sexual behavior are numerous in programming consumed by young people (Brown, 2002; Aubrey et al., 2021), and heterosexual identities are normalized through their abundance (Ward, 2003; Ward et al., 2014) and framed as the default (i.e., "compulsory heterosexuality," Rich, 2002). Alternatively, non-heterosexual identities in media and mediated representations of non-heterosexual interactions are novel and rare (Bond, 2014) but are frequently used by young people to understand feelings of attraction to members of the same gender.

However, messages identified by researchers and the interpretation of media content by audiences are different constructs (Ahuvia, 2001), and this disparity becomes even more glaring in the current media environment. Gen Z audiences (born 1997-2012) – simultaneously eager to understand the world around them as emerging adults and isolated from real-world social interactions during the start of the COVID-19 pandemic in early 2020 – relied on media during an important developmental period, but their interpretations of media messages regarding sex and sexuality have not often been investigated.

In fall of 2021, a cohort of 458 first-year college students provided their favorite media content across a wide variety of platforms and genres and

DOI: 10.4324/9781032648880-7

critically considered how social categories like race, gender, and sexuality were represented as part of the "Home College Experience" (HCE), a short media literacy course that featured a diversity and inclusion focused curriculum for professional communication students. Through systematic inquisition and assessment, the current chapter reveals how a cross section of first-year college students makes sense of messages regarding sexuality in some of their favorite media content, thus illuminating how the current media landscape impacts late adolescents.

Sensemaking

Sensemaking refers to the processes by which individuals make sense of events through processing information from other people's interpretations, understandings, and reactions to said events (Dervin, 1983). Sensemaking involves two processes: collecting data and framing data (Klein et al., 2006). Reflecting on familiar messages and considering them through the lens of social justice and marginalization can foster constructivist learning that "emphasizes the agency of the learning … [by arranging] challenging experiences in order to accelerate the change process" (Suthers, 2006 p. 316).

The HCE program guided students through a series of media literacy activities wherein they considered their own (mediated) experiences and constructed a more robust understanding and interpretation of their favorite content. Whereas sensemaking often relies on intersubjectivity, or "the coordinated moment-to-moment interaction of embodied agents and agents' experience of this process" (Fuchs & de Jaegher, 2009, p. 482), the HCE relied on intra-subjectivity, or the coordinated moment-to-moment interaction of one's embodiment across time, where a *single* participant contributes to a composition of interrelated interpretations.

Receiver-Oriented Message Analysis (ROMA)

Receiver-oriented message analysis (ROMA) addresses gaps in content analyses methodology that do not account for how messages are received. Researchers often neglect to "consult receivers to obtain realistic assessments of content as it is actually perceived by particular types of audiences" (Austin, 2010, p. 195). Introduced by Austin et al. (2007), ROMA systematically probes message receivers to "reveal their own content-based perceptions" (p. 96), using quantitative measures to assess qualitative and nuanced responses within different groups (Austin, 2010).

However, even these studies rarely grab moment-to-moment investigations of this process, making the HCE a rare opportunity to assess college students' understanding and interpretation of mediated sexuality. The

HCE program is not a formal ROMA study as students did not systematically analyze the same media artifacts. However, in the spirit of ROMA, students documented their interpretations of media messages, providing a large-scale qualitative corpus about how college students "construct sense" (Dervin, 1983, p. 7).

The Home College Experience (HCE)

The current analyses are drawn from data collected in Fall 2021 during HCE. All 458 incoming first-year students received credit for completing the program, which included three activities that explored their relationship with media. Each activity was followed by a structured small group discussion of 12–16 students with one faculty or staff member serving as instructor that featured anonymized and aggregated student responses.

Students first listed their favorite content (e.g., book, movie, television show, musician, influencer) in Activity 1 (n = 391) and indicated which of these media they use to connect with others and understand themselves. Activity 2 (n = 432) featured an exercise from Holtzman and Sharpe (2014) that was adapted from content analysis methods. The analyses in this chapter are taken from the second activity, and further details are provided below. Students applied these lessons in Activity 3 (n = 275) by conducting semi-structured interviews with individuals with whom they were demographically different on multiple categories.

Post hoc approval was obtained by the university's Office of Research Integrity and Protections as archival content associated with a course. Students were aware that their responses would be shared in the discussion without identifiers and received their responses to the activities via email. However, some students may have avoided sharing certain observations or reactions given the classroom setting; therefore, the findings associated with this corpus should be considered a conservative representation of students' observations.

Activity 2: Analyzing messages in media

Students selected an artifact from their list of favorite content and described its general messages before reading a selection that describes the importance of representing race, class, gender, and sexuality in entertainment media (Holtzman & Sharpe, 2014). Students then indicated the extent to which race, ethnicity, gender, sexuality, socioeconomic class, and ability were present in their targeted content using a four-point scale (i.e., not present, present but minor, significant, or outstanding); sexuality was defined as follows: "A person's sexual orientation, or the category of people that someone is attracted to physically or emotionally relative to their gender, and the resulting identity." Students who indicated "not present" elaborated the composition of characters; students who indicated "present but minor" elaborated how the construct was addressed and ignored; and students who indicated "significant" or "outstanding" elaborated how the content made them think *differently* about the content (for specific wording, see Figure 5.1).

Targeted content

Students selected a wide array of media types ranging across time and including older books like *Pride and Prejudice* (1813), *The Great Gatsby* (1925), and *Rebecca* (1938) to current television shows like *The Boys* (2019), *Dave* (2020), and *The Premise* (2021), as well as popular franchises, including Harry Potter and Marvel movies.[1] Television shows were the most popular (27.8%), followed by musicians (18.2%), movies (16%), news outlets (11.2%), books (7.0%), podcasts (5.4%), influencers (4.2%), and magazines (2.6%). The most popular content targeted included ESPN ($n = 17$; news, television show, radio), Harry Styles ($k = 9$; musician), Taylor Swift ($k = 9$; musician), and *The New York Times* ($k = 9$; news). Some students analyzed social media platforms, but many of these responses addressed platform affordances without mentioning specific content. Therefore, these responses were dropped from the following analyses, resulting in a final $N = 312$.

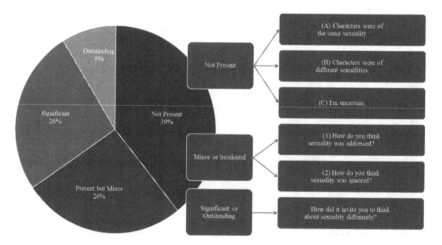

FIGURE 5.1   Student responses to initial question of whether the topic of sexuality was present in their targeted media content and associated progression of items; more than 90% of students provided an open-ended response.

Student demographics

Although this research features a selection of responses from the second activity, demographic information was collected from a different subsample during the third activity; this is reported for context but will not be deployed in the current analyses. The average age was 18.27 years (SD = .580).[2] Almost two-thirds of the sample identified as women (61.1%), 35.6% identified as men, seven identified as nonbinary, one as a trans woman, and two preferred not to say. The majority identified as White or of European descent (78.1%); 4.2% identified as Black or of African descent, 3.6% identified as Asian or of Asian descent, 5.6% identified as Latine, and 3.9% identified as mixed. Almost all (95.4%) were born in the United States. Four-fifths (81%) identified as heterosexual, 12.1% identified as bisexual or pansexual, 2.3% identified as gay, 2.3% as another sexuality, and 2.3% preferred not to say. Regarding socioeconomic class[3], 57.8% self-identified as middle, 33% identified as upper, 5.6% identified as lower, and 3.6% preferred not to say. Finally, almost one-third (32.6%) identified as living with one or more disabilities.

Analysis and findings

Representation of sexuality varied widely. More than one-third (39%) indicated that discussion of sexuality was not present in the content they chose to analyze, 26.2% indicated that discussions of sexuality were present but minor, 25.6% indicated that these topics were significant, and 8.9% stated that they were outstanding.[4] Open-ended responses were then subjected to thematic analysis (Braun & Clark, 2006), a widely used methodology in qualitative psychology, where researchers identify themes in attitudes and behaviors through systematically analyzing interviews and other user-generated content. First, the lead investigator read the student responses clustered by prompt (see Figure 5.1) to become familiar with the data and generated a series of initial codes. The responses were then re-read to fine-tune the initial codes, highlight pertinent examples, and aggregate the codes into themes (see Figure 5.2). These themes were then reviewed, defined, named, and presented.

Heterosexuality is normalized

Students frequently acknowledged that sexuality was a spectrum that varied infinitely, but many responses focused on whether non-heterosexual identities were present, thus normalizing heterosexuality through two related but distinct ways: (1) implicitly: students did not consider representations of heterosexuality when asked whether sexuality was present in their media, and

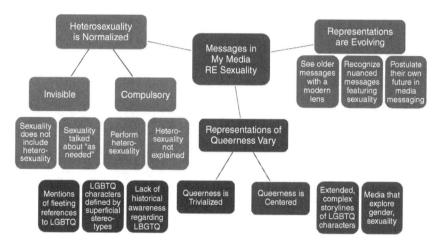

FIGURE 5.2 Developed thematic map showing three main themes.

Note: Themes and related subthemes are grouped by color.

(2) explicitly: students acknowledged that heterosexual relationships consti-
tuted a representation of sexuality even if it was unspoken.

Heterosexuality is invisible

Of the students who indicated that sexuality was absent from their media,
more than half (53.4%) reported that the content was composed entirely
of heterosexual or straight characters.[5] In other words, approximately one-
fifth of *all* students indicated that heterosexual representation did not qual-
ify as "representing sexuality." Much like discussions of Whiteness with
respect to race (Dyer, 2005), maleness with respect to gender (Connell &
Messerschmidt, 2005), or middle-class with respect to socioeconomic class
(Manstead, 2018), the hegemonically dominant category often goes unno-
ticed and unexplored.

This normalization of heterosexuality was also evident in students'
opinions regarding when and where sexuality should be discussed – or that
queer sexualities should be largely invisible or closeted. They acknowledged that sexuality was addressed "as needed" or "as necessary"; sexuality was discussed if a story featured someone with a marginalized sexual
identity or during Pride month (e.g., "For pride month, *The View* offers
daily facts and accomplishments of the LGBTQ+ community to their lis-
teners … Yet, none of the current hosts identify with the community").
Outside of these instances, students did not see messages that actively
engaged with conversations about sexuality – heterosexual or queer – and
instead rationalized the absence of any deeper discussion. In the television

show *Survivor*, "Sexuality is addressed when contestants reveal it – the show won't go out of its way to talk about it"; discussions of sexuality on *The Today Show* occur "during hard news stories whenever needed"; and Pat McAfee's podcast "is a football show, we don't need to know if you're LGBQT or straight." To address sexuality only when it is needed or "as necessary" maintains the implicit normativity of heterosexuality, in that non-heterosexual identities are considered addressing sexuality.

Heterosexuality is compulsory

Some students acknowledged that regardless of whether featured individuals were heterosexual, they would need to *appear* heterosexual to fit in. In line with the theory of "compulsory heterosexuality" (Rich, 2002, p. 11), students mentioned that they received messages that performances of heterosexuality were necessary (e.g., in *The Sopranos*, "it was viewed as bad if you didn't go with the social norms," most *Mamma Mia* characters "were straight or assumed to be straight"). Similarly, students reporting that sexuality was "present but minor" also acknowledged that heterosexual intimacy or relationships qualified (e.g., "She talks about her husband alot [sic], and their ideas of sexuality as it ties into the Mormon culture they grew up in") but rarely explicated how characters in heterosexual relationships addressed or ignored sexuality. Ultimately, students recognized that there were non-heterosexual identities and that people deserved respect regardless of their sexuality, but they did not share observations that rationalized the presentation of heterosexuality in a manner similar to queer identities.

Representations of queerness vary

Despite this pervasive interpretation of heterosexuality as normal, students shared a nuanced understanding of sexuality that affected their interpretations of media messages. Many students who indicated that their targeted media featured different types of sexualities (10.2% of those who said sexuality was not present) or who were uncertain (36.4% of those who said sexuality was not present) acknowledged that sexuality was *not* overt (e.g., in the book *Just Mercy*, "Sexuality was not explicitly addressed, so I can't assume who identified in what ways"). Similarly, many students reported that they saw a wide array of representations of queerness in their media, ranging from trivialization to celebration.

Queerness is trivialized

Students described any mention of LGBTQ identities (e.g., Pride month playlists, someone coming out as LGBTQ, queer characters on television shows) as well as jokes at the expense of queer people (e.g., On *Seinfeld*, "it was occasionally joked about in passing while also taking the stance that there is nothing wrong with being non-heterosexual" and "a few homophobic slurs" in the movie *Goodfellas*), among the 26.2% of students who indicated that sexuality was present but minor. Students also mentioned instances when queer characters were used as secondary characters (e.g., *How I Met Your Mother* addressed the LGBTQ community "through side characters and in casual conversation" but were not foregrounded in any of the main characters or narratives) or as tools to advance the narrative of the main (heterosexual) characters (e.g., several students mentioned Ross' ex-wife on the sitcom *Friends* who left him when she came out as a lesbian).

When queer characters were foregrounded, students described observing a focus on their "appearance, style, and personal qualities" (Lind & Salo, 2002, p. 217), trivializing them and often reinforcing stereotypes. Students called these artifacts out for perpetuating a collective misunderstanding of the experience and diversity of queerness. Students lamented the one gay character in *The Office*, whose "experiences are poked fun at throughout the show," how queerness was used for "comedic purposes only" on *How I Met Your Mother*, and on *New Girl*, "Jess had two lesbian friends … And Megan Fox's character in the last 2 seasons was bisexual, which was super fetishized and misrepresented." Even though they considered these programs among their favorites, they were not beyond reproach. Some students expressed frustration that these minor representations were performative, an outcome of what they believed to be the producers' need to "check that box."

Some students justified representations of sexuality that may appear problematic. This approach simultaneously worked to trivialize conversations about sexuality in general and rationalize corporate decisions. In the worst cases, there was a lack of historical awareness that indicates much more insidious effects of non-recognition. A small but striking minority of students dismissed the lack of representation because queerness simply didn't exist (e.g., *Monty Python and the Holy Grail* "was released in 1975, which was prior to much of the conversation about LGBTQIA+ and the community that is present today"; *Ferris Bueller's Day Off* featured "no other sexualities, mainly because it wasn't very common to be anything other than heterosexual in the 80s"). These defensive strategies worked to trivialize queerness by avoiding a deeper critical conversation about representation and societal effects. In some cases, students appeared to defuse or deflect any lack of robust discussion by amplifying seemingly small actions taken by their favorite musician (e.g., Harry Styles "runs around" with a pride flag) or influencers (e.g., Emma Chamberlain "discusses her support for the LGBT+ community briefly," basketball influencer D'vontay Friga "does not discriminate").

Queerness is centered

Over one-third of students said that sexuality was significant or outstanding in their selected content, many of which described open discussions about sexuality and specifically marginalized sexualities. These students described extended storylines about a character's sexuality and the associated experiences. They mentioned that LGBTQ people engaging in storylines did not emphasize their sexuality and extended critical queer readings of content and production considerations (e.g., *Us*). Students also expressed learning about – and advocating for – a spectrum of sexualities (Taylor Swift "has many songs targeting and calling out homophobia, and is a huge advocate for LGBTQ rights"). Contrasted with earlier mentions of seemingly "trivial" instances of representation or advocacy, these students described observing extended and nuanced messages about sexuality in their favorite media, not just fleeting moments.

Furthermore, contrary to stereotypical representations of queer identities described in earlier research, several students expressed that queerness was not synonymous with (hyper)sexuality nor was it condemned. There was content that had sexual themes or were sexually explicit (e.g., *Sex and the City, Game of Thrones*), but few students chose to describe messages that were particularly focused on sexual activities. Many of the targeted musicians produce what is widely considered to be sexually charged content but students read this content as content that represented their nuanced identity with gender and sexuality and how they advocated for marginalized communities, including queer artists like Doja Cat who "claims her own sexuality (bi), while also sexualizing herself in a powerful way," and heterosexual artists like Playboi Carti, who "doesn't see what he wears as an indicator of his sexual preference, but rather his fashion preference."

Representations of sexuality are evolving

Students exhibited a critical sensibility and robust engagement with issues of sexuality, recognizing that sexuality was both a conservative product of prior generations as well as a progressive and complex construct evident through their interpersonal upbringing and societal influence. Furthermore, they noted that their favorite media content does not always feature robust representation of this spectrum, including past and present content, reading past content through a contemporary lens as well as a historical one.

Sitcoms of the nineties and noughties like *Friends, The Sopranos, How I Met Your Mother, Gilmore Girls, The Office*, and *Gossip Girl* were simultaneously lauded and scrutinized. Multiple students recognized that *Friends* was notoriously poor when representing issues of sexuality regarding Ross' ex-wife, Carol, and gender regarding Chandler's parent Charles/Helena who transitioned, but students often dismissed these instances as artifacts of their time.[6] In *How I Met Your Mother*, multiple students described a satirical reading of the character and narratives of Barney Stimson, a "crazy sex-driven heterosexual male," who was played by Neil Patrick Harris, who is openly gay.

Even though many students associated topics of sexuality with non-heterosexual identities, students recognized that one should not simply assume a character to be heterosexual if it is not made evident, although few explicitly mentioned that not mentioning sexuality implied heterosexuality. They also acknowledged the preponderance of heterosexuality as an entrenched social norm that deserved resistance, and they recognized when it was done with care: ESPN "did a good job covering NFL player Carl Nassib coming out as gay"; "guests have come out with their sexuality on the air or have discussed what it's been like to discover their feelings on their own sexuality" on the *Joe Rogan Experience* podcast; and *Schitt's Creek* writers "intentionally created a setting where queer characters didn't have to experience fear surrounding their sexuality and they could live and love just as the straight characters do." This diversity of narratives allowed their content to simultaneously respect people's boundaries while vicariously and voyeuristically observing personal journeys.

Many students described what they liked in media content, thereby postulating what a robust representation of sexuality would look like in future media messages. They posited media content that normalizes diverse sexual identities through queer characters who could be free of stereotypical anti-queer expectations (e.g., "*Glee* had several characters of varying sexualities with complex relationships and character traits"). Students also observed ambiguity in their media messages as a means of disrupting discourse and inviting the audience (and by extension themselves) to think about sexuality in new ways: they described that Elton John's music lacked gender specificity, a sexually ambiguous character in the first few seasons of *It's Always Sunny in Philadelphia* was met with acceptance when they came out; and the book *Conversations with Friends* (2017) features a bisexual protagonist that one student appreciated because it "invites the reader to consider sexuality."

Discussion

The current analysis provides a nuanced perspective of how Gen Z college students make sense of sexuality in their favorite media content using a corpus of subjective interpretations across a wide array of content and observers made possible by the HCE exercise, resulting in a somewhat paradoxical approach to media analysis (Ahuvia, 2001). Even though Gen Z are considered to be one of the most progressive generations regarding sexuality and gender, 20.8% of Gen Z adults identify as LGBTQ (Jones, 2022) and more than half (59%) believe that there should be more than two gender options on forms (Kenney, 2020), students reported that heterosexuality was still normalized, queerness was both trivialized and centered, and representations of sexuality were still evolving in their favorite media.

In 2021, 18- and 19-year-old college students recognize the spectrum of sexuality and are realistic about its representation in their favorite media content. Some students approached messages with a critical lens and were eager to consider their role in future representations, whereas others – despite recognizing limited representation – observed and rationalized hegemonically heterosexual content. Although social media can disrupt expectations of sexuality because of the unique opportunity for users to share stories independent of industry gatekeepers, morality codes, or social conventions, Gen Z audiences are still engaging with, learning from, and critically probing content that presents both conservative and complex representations of sexuality, demanding greater consideration of their varied media use and the nuanced knowledge they bring to interpreting these messages.

Notes

1 When considering the publication, release, and premiere dates of books, movies, and television shows ($k = 140$; 44.8%), the average year of publication was 2001 ($SD = 22.91$).

2 Students indicating that they were 17 years old or younger were removed from the entire dataset.

3 If students were uncertain, they were forwarded to the Pew Research Income Calculator (Bennett et al., 2020), but this distribution is notoriously unreliable (Wenger & Zaber, 2021), especially with respect to a student population.

4 Half of students who analyzed television shows ($\chi^2 = 9.947$, $p = .001$) and musicians ($\chi^2 = 14.231$, $p < .001$) said that sexuality was discussed in a significant or outstanding manner. This was a significantly higher percentage compared to students who analyzed other mediums: only a quarter of students who analyzed books, podcasts, and news outlets as well as less than 10% of students who analyzed movies or influencers said that their targeted content addressed sexuality in a significant or outstanding manner.

5 There were no instances of all characters/actors in a given media being all gay or all lesbian.

6 No student mentioned these characters by name; they were only mentioned relative to the heterosexual lead.

References

Ahuvia, A. (2001). Traditional, interpretive, and reception based content analyses: Improving the ability of content analysis to address issues of pragmatic and theoretical concern. *Social Indicators Research, 54*, 139–172. https://doi.org/10.1023/A:1011087813505

Aubrey, J. S., Dajches, L., & Terán, L. (2021). Media as a source of sexual socialization for emerging adults. In L. Dajches, L. Terán, & J. S. Aubrey (Eds.) *Sexuality in Emerging Adulthood*. Oxford University Press. https://doi.org/10.1093/oso/9780190057008.003.0019

Austin, E. W. (2010). Receiver-oriented message analysis: Lessons from alcohol advertising. In A. Jordan, D. Kunkel, J. Mangalnello, & M. Fishbein (Eds.), *Media Messages and Public Health* (pp. 210–228). Routledge.

Austin, E. W., Pinkleton, B. E., Hust, S. J. T., & Miller, A. C. R. (2007). The locus of message meaning: Differences between trained coders and untrained message recipients in the analysis of alcoholic beverage advertising. *Communication Methods and Measures, 1*(2), 91–111. https://doi.org/10.1080/19312450701399354

Bennett, J., Fry, R., & Kochhar, R. (2020, July 23). *Are you in the American middle class? Find out with our income calculator*. Pew Research Center. https://www.pewresearch.org/short-reads/2020/07/23/are-you-in-the-american-middle-class/.

Bond, B. J. (2014). Sex and sexuality in entertainment media popular with lesbian, gay, and bisexual adolescents. *Mass Communication and Society, 17*(1), 98–120. https://doi.org/10.1080/15205436.2013.816739.

Braun, V., & Clarke, V. (2006). Using thematic analysis in psychology. *Qualitative Research in Psychology, 3*(2), 77–101. https://doi.org/10.1191/1478088706qp063oa

Brown, J. D. (2002). Mass media influences on sexuality. *The Journal of Sex Research, 39*(1), 42–45. https://doi.org/10.1080/00224490209552118

Connell, R. W., & Messerschmidt, J. W. (2005). Hegemonic masculinity: Rethinking the concept. *Gender & Society, 19*(6), 829–859. https://doi.org/10.1177/0891243205278639

Dervin, B. (1983). An overview of sense-making research: Concepts, methods and results. Paper presented at the annual meeting of the International Communication Association, Dallas, TX, May. [On-line]. http://communication.sbs.ohio-state.edu/sense-making/art/artdervin83.html

Dyer, R. (2005). The matter of whiteness. In P. Rothenberg (Ed.), *White privilege: Essential readings on the other side of racism* (pp. 9–14). Worth Publishing.

Fuchs, T., & De Jaegher, H. (2009). Enactive intersubjectivity: Participatory sense-making and mutual incorporation. *Phenomenology and the Cognitive Sciences, 8*(4), 465–486. https://doi.org/10.1007/s11097-009-9136-4

Holtzman, L., & Sharpe, L. (2014). *Media Messages: What film, television, and popular music teach us about race, class, gender, and sexual orientation*. Routledge. https://doi.org/10.4324/9781315702469

Jones, J. M. (2022, February 17). LGBT identification in U.S. ticks up to 7.1%. *Gallup*. https://news.gallup.com/poll/389792/lgbt-identification-ticks-up.aspx

Kenney, J. (2020, April 8). Companies can't ignore shifting gender norms. *Harvard Business Review*. https://hbr.org/2020/04/companies-cant-ignore-shifting-gender-norms

Klein, G., Moon, B., & Hoffman, R. R. (2006). Making sense of sensemaking 1: Alternative perspectives. *IEEE intelligent systems, 21*(4), 70–73. https://doi.org/10.1109/MIS.2006.75

Lind, R. A., & Salo, C. (2002). The framing of feminists and feminism in news and public affairs programs in U.S. electronic media. *Journal of Communication, 52*(1), 211–228.https://doi.org/10.1111/j.1460-2466.2002.tb02540.x

Manstead, A. S. (2018). The psychology of social class: How socioeconomic status impacts thought, feelings, and behaviour. *British Journal of Social Psychology, 57*(2), 267–291. https://doi.org/10.1111/bjso.12251

Rich, A. (2002). Compulsory heterosexuality and lesbian existence. In P. Aggleton & R. Parker (Eds.), *Culture, Society and Sexuality* (pp. 199–225). Routledge. https://doi.org/10.4324/9780203020173

Suthers, D. D. (2006). Technology affordances for intersubjective meaning making: A research agenda for CSCL. *International Journal of Computer-supported Collaborative Learning, 1*, 315–337.

Ward, L. M. (2003). Understanding the role of entertainment media in the sexual socialization of American youth: A review of empirical research. *Developmental Review, 23*(3), 347–388. https://doi.org/10.1016/S0273-2297(03)00013-3

Ward, L. M., Reed, L., Trinh, S. L., & Foust, M. (2014). Sexuality and entertainment media. In D. L. Tolman, L. M. Diamond, J. A. Bauermeister, W. H. George, J. G. Pfaus, & L. M. Ward (Eds.), *APA handbook of sexuality and psychology, Vol. 2. Contextual approaches* (pp. 373–423). American Psychological Association. https://doi.org/10.1037/14194-012

Wenger, J. B., & Zaber, M. A. (2021). *Who is middle class?* RAND. https://www.rand.org/pubs/perspectives/PEA1141-3.html.

6

LGBTQ YOUTH REPORT ON MEDIA-BASED INTERACTIONS WITH THEIR PARENTS

Marie-Louise Mares and Yuchi Anthony Chen

Media representations and online communities serve important functions for lesbian, gay, bisexual, transgender, and queer (LGBTQ) communities, including identity exploration and support (e.g., Bond, 2018; Ybarra et al., 2015). Repeated exposure to positive depictions of LGBTQ characters and experiences may also reduce prejudice and increase understanding among cisgender, heterosexual viewers (e.g., Bond, 2021; Schiappa et al., 2006). The current chapter examines whether media depictions may help families with LGBTQ teens have conversations about the teen's sexual orientation and/or gender.

Although parental support is one of the strongest predictors of LGBTQ youths' mental health (Milton & Knutson, 2023), families often struggle to communicate effectively in this context. A review of research on parent–teen sex communication with sexual and gender minority youth found that teens wanted their parents to discuss sex but were dissatisfied with the depth and breadth of such conversations (McKay & Fontenot, 2020). Other studies find variation in parental support and communication: some parents respond to their children coming out with love and support, others give ambivalent, invalidating, or even hostile responses (e.g., van Bergen et al., 2021), including (in some instances) physical violence (Galop, 2022).

Media content may potentially facilitate family conversations about youth identities, although most research has focused on other domains. For example, surveys of U.S. Black parents indicate that they discuss news reports of anti-Black police violence with their children (e.g., Sullivan et al., 2021), critique stereotypical entertainment depictions, and encourage viewing that would foster their child's sense of racial identity and

DOI: 10.4324/9781032648880-8

prepare their child for racial bias (McClain & Mares, 2021). In other work, youths' media exposure led them to talk with their parents about their political (e.g., McDevitt, 2005) and religious (Boyatzis & Janicki, 2003) beliefs. Fewer scholars have examined media-elicited family discussions of LGBTQ identities, but LGBTQ youth and adults report that their parents' exposure to relevant media depictions helped their parents accept their sexual orientation (Samarova et al., 2014) and understand the LGBTQ community more broadly (GLAAD, 2021).

We began our own work in this area by surveying two samples of U.S. LGBTQ 18- and 19-year-olds (Mares et al., 2022) and then a sample of U.S. LGBTQ 13- to 17-year-olds and one of their parents (Mares et al., 2023), asking about the frequency and emotional tone of family interactions about LGBTQ media depictions. For both parents and teens, the positivity of these moments was associated with ratings of parental support for the teen's sexual or gender identity (Mares et al., 2022, 2023). Because those papers were focused on teens' and parents' use of specific socialization strategies (i.e., encouraging, restricting, critiquing identity-related media content) and on the implications for identity support, we did not probe the details of their media-inspired conversations. In the current chapter, we re-analyze data from the two samples of 18- and 19-year-olds (Mares et al., 2022), focusing in more detail on (a) their ratings of how often LGBTQ-oriented media led them to discuss specific topics with their parents, and (b) their open-ended descriptions of media-based interactions with their parents. The goal was to provide more insight into these conversations.

The current sample

We recruited two samples of LGBTQ teens aged 18 and 19 from two online panels (MTurk, $n = 276$, and Qualtrics, $n = 369$) to complete an online survey. As approved by the IRB at the authors' institution, all teens gave written consent to participate; they were old enough not to need parental consent. For details of the survey and procedure, see Mares et al. (2022).

After excluding 38 participants who missed items for the measure of media-inspired discussions, the combined sample totaled $N = 607$. At the start of the survey, participants selected one LGBTQ identity to focus on for the survey, which then auto-filled subsequent items. Sample demographics are given in Table 6.1.

Quantitative ratings of media-elicited discussions

Teens rated how often identity-related media content led them to discuss seven topics with their parents. As shown in Table 6.1, teens reported that

TABLE 6.1 Demographics, measurements, and descriptive statistics

	Percent	n
Race/Ethnicity (Check all that apply)		
American Indian or Alaskan Native	1.32	8
Asian or Asian American	7.41	45
Black or African American	11.86	72
Hawaiian or Pacific Islander	0.16	1
Hispanic or Latino/Latina/Latinx	10.05	61
Mixed Race/Ethnicity	9.88	60
White	58.32	354
Other	0.99	6
Sexual Orientation (Check all that apply)		
Straight	4.78	29
Lesbian (focal identity $n = 101$)	20.10	122
Gay (focal identity $n = 72$)	15.32	93
Bisexual (focal identity $n = 343$)	56.84	345
Queer (focal identity $n = 26$)	9.39	57
Other	6.59	40
Gender Identity (Check all that apply)		
Cisgender Female	58.65	356
Cisgender Male	17.79	108
Transgender Female (either transgender focal identity $n = 35$)	6.26	38
Transgender Male	6.76	41
Gender Nonbinary (focal identity $n = 30$)	1.54	64

	M	(SD)
Frequency of Media-Inspired Discussion (1 never, 5 very often)		
Sexual risk related to being (selected identity)	2.34	(1.36)
Not being ashamed of being (selected identity)	2.48	(1.37)
Being proud to be (selected identity)	2.54	(1.39)
Discriminations faced by those who are (selected identity)	2.57	(1.34)
Mental health risks (like depression) related to being (selected identity)	2.58	(1.37)
What it means to be (selected identity)	2.63	(1.39)
Equal rights (like marriage, bathroom choices)	2.88	(1.41)

Note: Focal identity refers to the identities that participants choose to focus on for quantitative measurements. Question stem for media-inspired topics: "How often, if ever, have movies, TV shows, or programs on streaming services like Netflix and Hulu prompted discussions between you and your parent(s) about the following topics?"

media had most often led to a discussion about equal rights but led less often to discussions of sexual risks, not feeling ashamed of, or being proud of, their LGBTQ identity.

To explore these patterns, we used latent profile analysis (LPA), which can uncover groupings (e.g., of individuals or items) based on combinations of variables (Oberski, 2016). LPA was conducted using the *MplusAutomation* package in R (Hallquist & Wiley, 2018), to analyze teens' ratings of how often media had inspired conversations about each topic. Based on the criteria recommended by Nylund-Gibson et al. (2019), the evaluation of models ranging from one to four profiles revealed that a three-profile model exhibited the optimal fit, characterized by low Bayesian Information Criterion and high entropy.

As Figure 6.1 shows, there was a low-engaging group in which parents and teens almost never discussed any of the topics in response to media (*n* = 229, 38%), a moderate-engaging group that sometimes did (*n* = 225, 37%), and a small, high-engaging group (*n* = 153, 25%) that did so relatively often, particularly for topics of pride and equal rights. The frequency of discussing sexual risk was consistently low in all three groups and equal rights was consistently high. The qualitative data provide some insights into these media-based interactions.

The qualitative prompts

We asked teens whether they could recall "a specific movie, TV show, or program featuring a [focal identity] individual" that they liked watching

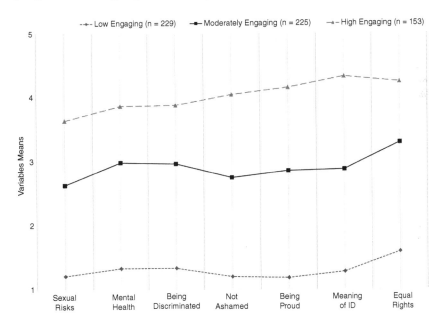

FIGURE 6.1   Item means for the three-profile model of media-inspired topics.

Note: Means reflect the frequency of participants' reported engagement with each media-inspired topic in each profile.

with their parent and to explain "what was it and what made it enjoyable to watch together." Those who only had negative experiences were asked, "Could you give an example and say what was negative about the situation?" Those who had never co-viewed read, "There could be lots of reasons why – it would be great if you could try to explain your situation a bit." Later, they were asked if they could think of specific content that had (among other things) "sparked a discussion with your parent about being [identity]? What was that content? ... If you've never done any of these things, it would be really helpful if you could explain why." The instructions stated that they could skip these questions.

Coding the qualitative responses

Only 63.1% of the sample ($n = 383$) gave qualitative answers that could be coded. The remaining 36.9% ($n = 224$) of teens gave very brief answers (e.g., listed a show but didn't elaborate) or left the open-ended questions blank, or wrote in nonsense/unclear answers. We initially interpreted these brief or non-answers as likely reflecting infrequent media-based interactions. However, there was no difference between those whose answers were categorized versus those not in their quantitative ratings of how often they and their parents had media-inspired discussion of the specific topics: $t(605) = 2.317$, $p = .156$ for the overall mean frequency of discussions, nor were there significant differences by teens' focal identity $\chi^2(5) = 10.411$, $p = .064$.

For the most part, teens' open-ended answers did not describe specific topics of conversations, focusing more on reasons for not having such interactions or on the affective tone of interactions when they did occur.

Reasons for infrequent media-based interactions related to LGBTQ identity

After examining the themes that emerged in teens' explanations for not having such interactions, we coded (0 no, 1 yes) whether teens said that they tended not to co-view or discuss identity-related content with their parents because (1) they feared negative responses and/or they perceived it would be too awkward or uncomfortable, (2) they perceived there to be only few and/or stigmatizing media depictions of their identity, or (3) pragmatic reasons, such as lack of time. These codes were not mutually exclusive. Krippendorff's alpha for the reliability of intercoder agreement between the two authors was above .90 for all three reasons. Table 6.2 gives the frequencies for each, within the overall sample and for each family profile. The two quotes below illustrate these different reasons,

TABLE 6.2 Coding teens' descriptions of media-based interactions with parents about being LGBTQ

	Differences by Family Latent Profile				
	Overall %	Low %	Moderate %	High %	χ^2
Reasons for Not Co-Viewing/Discussing With Parents					
Negative/Awkward ($n = 84$)	13.8	23.1$_a$	8.9$_b$	7.2$_b$	26.93***
Pragmatic Obstacles ($n = 58$)	9.6	16.6$_a$	6.2$_b$	3.9$_b$	21.64***
Inadequate Depictions ($n = 49$)	8.1	12.7$_a$	7.1$_{ab}$	2.6$_b$	12.93**
Affective Tone of Interaction					
Positive ($n = 180$)	29.7	16.2$_b$	38.7$_a$	36.6$_a$	32.30***
Negative ($n = 105$)	17.3	21.0	16.0	13.7	3.87

Notes: **$p < .01$, ***$p < .001$.

including their co-occurrence. (Brackets contain family profile and teens' focal identity.)

> I have never intentionally watched a show with queer characters in it with my parents. They are conservative Christians and I'm in the closet. Sometimes I'll show them movies that I really like and they'll happen to have queer characters but I'm very uncomfortable and overly self-conscious when these come on so I don't usually show these to my parents.
>
> *[low, queer]*

> I haven't watched any programs featuring a transgender character. For one thing, it's difficult to even find shows or movies that have a trans character in there, especially a trans man. Furthermore, my parents wouldn't be very open to watching this kind of thing and it would feel very forced to have them watch it with me. Additionally, we don't watch much of anything together because it's so difficult to find common interests and it's hard for me to be around them sometimes.
>
> *[low, transgender]*

As shown in Table 6.2, teens in the low-engaging group were significantly more likely to mention each of these three reasons than teens in high-engaging and moderate-engaging families. We also tested whether the percentage of teens reporting each reason varied by the teen's focal identity. Given the small numbers of queer, transgender, and nonbinary youth, we present these exploratory findings with caution. A higher percentage of transgender teens (34.3%) than gay (12.5%) and bisexual (10.5%) teens mentioned negative/awkward interactions with their parents, while other groups didn't differ, χ^2 (1) = 18.50, p < .01. Similarly, a higher percentage of transgender teens (22.9%) than gay (4.2%), lesbian (5.9%), and bisexual (7.3%) teens mentioned that the media included inadequate depictions of their identity, while other groups didn't differ, χ^2 (1) = 19.07, p < .05.

Emotional tone of media-inspired interactions about LGBTQ identity

For those youth who did describe a media-based interaction related to their LGBTQ identity, we coded whether it was described as positive and/or negative. Krippendorff's alpha for intercoder reliability was above .90 for both codes.

Positive interactions

About 30% of teens described some positive aspect of a media-based interaction related to their identity (see Table 6.2). Some emphasized the fun, bonding aspects of co-viewing specific shows, such as *RuPaul's Drag Race*, a reality competition show featuring drag queens.

> We love the fashion and the drama. It also keeps us in touch!
>
> *[moderate, gay]*

Others appreciated when their parents reacted to depictions of same-sex physical intimacy just as they did to depictions of heterosexual intimacy, as in the example below of responses to a TV series depicting the lives of young adults in New York City.

> I watched *Girls* with my mom where there's bisexual sexual activity sometimes. She reacts the same as with any heterosexual sexual scenes. She is completely accepting of it.
>
> *[high, bisexual]*

Finally, some teens reported that exposure to media content with a primary LGBTQ character (as in the film below about a teen gay romance) had helped their parents understand and/or support their identity.

Call Me by Your Name ... Thanks to this movie, my parents today accept I am being gay.

[moderate, gay]

Given the importance of media-inspired identity support, we systematically coded all such mentions and found 39 instances (6.4% of all teens). As such, increased support in response to a particular depiction was a relatively rare (although seemingly powerful) experience in our sample.

Teens in low-engaging families were less likely to describe a positive interaction than those in the moderate- and high-engaging families. Teens in the high-engaging group (who had given higher quantitative ratings to frequency of discussing seemingly positive topics like equality and pride) did not differ significantly from teens in the moderate-engaging group in the frequency of describing positive interactions. There were no significant differences in teens' focal LGBTQ identity.

Negative interactions

Approximately 17% of teen participants described a negative-media-based interaction with their parents. These included instances when the parent got angry at seeing LGBTQ representation and made hostile, even aggressive comments. The example below reflects the potential for parental physical violence, illustrating the Galop's (2022) findings about instances of physical abuse by parents of LGBTQ youth, particularly trans and nonbinary youth.

The Rocko movie on Netflix. he said he would "beat the shit" out of his child if they thought they were trans.

[low, transgender]

Some parents made a face in response to a scene of same-sex physical intimacy, stopped watching, or fast-forwarded scenes with LGBTQ characters.

I remember a while ago, perhaps a year, when I seen something on TV that featured a bisexual couple. I watched for my mother's reaction while watching, and she seemed ... almost disgusted. (ellipses in original). It made me feel terrible about myself, and that I would never be able to tell her about my sexuality.

[high, bisexual]

In some instances, media content elicited parents' religious objections or comments that same-sex relationships were immoral or unnatural. Finally, there were also instances where the teen had encouraged their parent to watch some identity-related content, but the parent did not watch.

> In … '*Steven Universe*', they introduce a character, Stevonnie that's non-binary and uses they/them pronouns. I encouraged my parents to watch this show not just because of this character but there is a lot of representation for gender queer and nonbinary characters. They brushed it off and never watched it.
>
> *[low, nonbinary]*

Mentions of negative-media-based interactions with parents did not differ significantly in frequency by family profile group or by teens' focal LGBTQ identity.

Discussion

There are three primary findings that we'd like to highlight. The first is the range and complexity of LGBTQ teens' experiences in co-viewing and discussing identity-related content with their parents. Again, we acknowledge the number of teens who did not provide reports, as well as other limitations of the sample. These were data from a narrow age range of teens living in the United States, and we did not probe intersections of LGBTQ identity with other identities, such as race and ethnicity, social class, or disability. Moreover, given that this was not a representative sample even of 18- and 19-year-old U.S. LGBTQ teens, the relative proportions of different experiences are less informative than the central finding of variation.

As illustrated in the LPA, some families almost never talked about LGBTQ-related issues in response to media content, some did so occasionally, and a smaller group did so fairly often. Some teens described moments of shared fun and pleasure while co-viewing, some reported media-inspired moments of feeling loved and understood, and others described parental disgust and hostility, particularly in response to depictions of physical intimacy. The sheer frequency or topic of conversations (as indicated by quantitative ratings and family profile) was not an indication of how positively these interactions were experienced. That is, although the low-engaging group reported fewer positive interactions, the moderate- and high-engaging groups didn't differ in this regard, and all three groups were as likely to describe a negative interaction. Nonetheless, codes for positive experiences outnumbered codes for negative experiences, suggesting that teens find more benefit than pain in such interactions.

Second, these findings reinforce the need for adequate media representations. This is nothing new: GLAAD has long been documenting the rise and fall of entertainment media representation of LGBTQ identities, including the intersections that are particularly lacking (GLAAD, 2023). However, the current findings suggest that co-viewing of identity-related media provides opportunities for parents to show their support and that symbolic annihilation of particular groups deprives them of those opportunities.

Third, teens' comments indicate the power of seemingly small moments in front of the screen. Parents' facial expressions and use of the remote, the comments they made, or their willingness to watch something recommended by their teen were used by teens as ways of diagnosing identity support. Parents may sometimes deliberately communicate their values and beliefs in such moments, but sometimes they may not fully recognize what they are conveying. Teens' accounts suggest that these interactions have emotional and relational consequences.

References

Bond, B. J. (2018). Parasocial relationships with media personae: Why they matter and how they differ among heterosexual, lesbian, gay, and bisexual adolescents. *Media Psychology*, *21*(3), 457–485. https://doi.org/10.1080/15213269.2017.1 416295

Bond, B. J. (2021). The development and influence of parasocial relationships with television characters: A longitudinal experimental test of prejudice reduction through parasocial contact. *Communication Research*, *48*(4), 573–593. https://doi.org/10.1177/0093650219900632

Boyatzis, C. J., & Janicki, D. L. (2003). Parent-child communication about religion: Survey and diary data on unilateral transmission and bi-directional reciprocity styles. *Review of Religious Research*, *44*(3), 252–270. https://doi.org/10.2307/3512386

Galop (2022). *LGBT+ Experiences of Abuse from Family Members*. https://galop.org.uk/wp-content/uploads/2022/04/Galop-LGBT-Experiences-of-Abuse-from-Family-Members.pdf

GLAAD (2021). *Where we are on TV 2020-2021*. https://glaad.org/whereweareontv20/

GLAAD (2023). *Where we are on TV 2023-2024*. https://glaad.org/whereweareontv23/

Hallquist, M. N., & Wiley, J. F. (2018). MplusAutomation: an R package for facilitating large-scale latent variable analyses in M plus. *Structural Equation Modeling: A Multidisciplinary Journal*, *25*(4), 621–638. https://doi.org/10.1080/107 05511.2017.1402334

Mares, M. L., Chen, Y. A., & Bond, B. J. (2023) Mutual socialization during media moments: U.S. LGBTQ teens and their parents negotiate identity support. *Journal of Communication*, *73*(2), 113–125. https://doi.org/10.1093/joc/jqac046

Mares, M. L., Chen, Y. A., & Bond, B. J. (2022). Mutual influence in LGBTQ teens' use of media to socialize their parents. *Media Psychology*, *25*(3), 441–468. https://doi.org/10.1080/15213269.2021.1969950

McClain, A. K., & Mares, M. L. (2021). Media messages: Intersections of ethnic-racial and media socialization in African American families. *Research in Human Development, 18*(4), 311–329. https://doi.org/10.1080/15427609.2021.2010491

McDevitt, M. (2005). The partisan child: Developmental provocation as a model of political socialization. *International Journal of Public Opinion Research, 18*(1), 67–88. https://doi.org/10.1093/ijpor/edh079

McKay, E. A., & Fontenot, H. B. (2020). Parent-adolescent sex communication with sexual and gender minority youth: An integrated review. *Journal of Pediatric Health Care, 34*(5), e37–e48. https://doi.org/10.1016/j.pedhc.2020.04.004

Milton, D. C., & Knutson, D. (2023). Family of origin, not chosen family, predicts psychological health in a LGBTQ+ sample. *Psychology of Sexual Orientation and Gender Diversity, 10*(2), 269–278. https://doi.org/10.1037/sgd0000531

Nylund-Gibson, K., Grimm, R. P., & Masyn, K. E. (2019). Prediction from latent classes: A demonstration of different approaches to include distal outcomes in mixture models. *Structural Equation Modeling: A Multidisciplinary Journal, 26*(6), 967–985. https://doi.org/10.1080/10705511.2019.1590146

Oberski, D. (2016). Mixture models: Latent profile and latent class analysis. In J. Robertson & M. Kaptein (Eds.), *Modern statistical methods for HCI* (pp. 275–287). Springer.

Samarova, V., Shilo, G., & Diamond, G. M. (2014). Changes in youths' perceived parental acceptance of their sexual minority status over time. *Journal of Research on Adolescence, 24*(4), 681–688. https://doi.org/10.1111/jora.12071

Schiappa, E., Gregg, P. B., & Hewes, D. E. (2006). Can one TV show make a difference? Will & Grace and the parasocial contact hypothesis. *Journal of Homosexuality, 51*(4), 15–37. https://doi.org/10.1300/J082v51n04_02

Sullivan, J. N., Eberhardt, J. L., & Roberts, S. O. (2021). Conversations about race in Black and White U.S. families: Before and after George Floyd's death. *Proceedings of the National Academy of Sciences, 118*(38), e2106366118. https://doi.org/10.1073/pnas.2106366118

van Bergen, D. D., Wilson, B. D., Russell, S. T., Gordon, A. G., & Rothblum, E. D. (2021). Parental responses to coming out by lesbian, gay, bisexual, queer, pansexual, or two-spirited people across three age cohorts. *Journal of Marriage and Family, 83*(4), 1116–1133. https://doi.org/10.1111/jomf.12731

Ybarra, M. L., Mitchell, K. J., Palmer, N. A., & Reisner, S. L. (2015). Online social support as a buffer against online and offline peer and sexual victimization among US LGBT and non-LGBT youth. *Child Abuse & Neglect, 39*, 123–136. https://doi.org/10.1016/j.chiabu.2014.08.006

7

GIRLS JUST WANNA … FIGURE OUT THEIR SEXUALITY

Exploring the Links between Celebrity Idolization and U.S. Adolescent Girls' Sexual Self-Concept

Leah Dajches, Larissa Terán, Kun Yan, and Jennifer Stevens Aubrey

Celebrity idols play a significant role in the emotional lives of many adolescents. Take international popstar Harry Styles, who had the fourth best-selling album in the United States in 2022 (Caulfield, 2023). His fan base is mostly made up of girls and young women, and he cultivates an exacting intimacy with them through his songs that speak to a frank interest in matters of sexual pleasure (Rosner, 2022). Styles is likely the object of romantic and sexual desire to many of his fans. To other fans, Styles might seem like a trusted friend, as his songs help fans process just about anything that relates to romantic relationships. His bold fashion choices signal to his fans that he is the "face of gender neutrality" (Khomami, 2022, para 9), whereas his "cheeky, chappy charm" (para 1) makes him seem like a fun friend to hang out with.

Styles aptly illustrates two main functions of celebrity for adolescents: a desirable romantic partner or a trusting friend (Tukachinsky, 2010). Both components are reflected in celebrity idolization, which is defined as devotion, involvement, or interest with a particular celebrity (Engle & Kasser, 2005). We contend that celebrity idolization is a way for adolescents to process emerging romantic and sexual feelings and experiences. For adolescent girls, in particular, developing an attachment with a celebrity idol can provide a way for them to imagine themselves in sexual relationships with desirable partners, even before they are ready to date in their real lives (Engle & Kasser, 2005; Karniol, 2001).

Celebrity idols are often associated with adolescent girls for several reasons. In addition to idols providing a convenient object for their emerging

DOI: 10.4324/9781032648880-9

romantic and sexual feelings, girls are socialized to believe that they should always be in love, and, because the relationship with a celebrity is often a one-way relationship (often called a parasocial relationship), girls likely feel safe and in control of managing these relationships (Karniol, 2001). Moreover, considering pervasive social stigma associated with adolescent girls' sexual behaviors (e.g., Kreager et al., 2016), there is more at stake for girls when they decide to engage in sexual behaviors (Walker et al., 2013). Thus, it behooves adolescent girls to explore and refine their romantic and sexual feelings before these feelings are put to the test in actual relationships. Therefore, our primary goal was to examine the relationship between adolescent girls' celebrity idolization and facets of their sexual self-concept. The emphasis in previous research is on *heterosexual* adolescent girls (Erickson & Dal Cin, 2018). However, given increased representation of lesbian, gay, bisexual, queer, and other diverse sexuality (LGBQ+) characters in the media (GLAAD, 2023), as well as more young people ("Generation Z") identifying as LGBQ+ (Jones, 2024), it is also important to understand the role of celebrity idolization in relation to the sexual self-concepts of LGBQ+ girls.

Celebrity idolization and adolescence

In today's media environment, digital media like social media affords adolescents various ways to engage with their favorite celebrity or influencer (e.g., following, liking/commenting on content). Through these interactions, and by consuming their idol's content, adolescents are supplied with values and information that help them figure out their identities (Greene & Adams-Price, 1990). Because adolescent girls are socialized to adhere to cultural norms and values of sexual restraint (Ehrenreich et al., 1992), one way that girls may explore their sexuality is through idolization. Idolizing a celebrity will likely not result in an actual relationship, and thus, idols are viewed as accessible and harmless targets for practicing one's developing sexual needs and feelings (Engle & Kasser, 2005).

Celebrity idolization often occurs at a romantic/sexual level. Indeed, celebrity attachments tend to form around the time that girls become aware of social norms that suggest that they should be interested in romance and sexuality (Erickson & Dal Cin, 2018). These celebrity attachments provoke adolescents to form unrealistic romantic beliefs and sexual expectations (Greene & Adams-Price, 1990; Karniol, 2001). For example, in a primarily heterosexual sample of late-adolescent women, romantic parasocial attachments to celebrities were related to higher levels of relationship-contingent self-esteem, stronger negative evaluations of their sexual experiences, and increased feelings of passionate love (Erickson &

Dal Cin, 2018). Likewise, among U.S. adolescents, romantic parasocial relationships with celebrities were associated with more idealized romantic beliefs (Tukachinsky & Dorros, 2018).

Conceptualizing the sexual self-concept

In adolescence, a major developmental task is sexual development, which includes important issues as to whom adolescents are attracted to and what they have to offer as a sexual partner (Rostosky et al., 2008). The latter is related to the development of a sexual self-concept (i.e., one's understanding of themselves within the sexual domain; Rostosky et al., 2008). Although dozens of studies have examined the influences of media exposure on adolescents' sexual socialization, which includes attitudes, norms, and expectations regarding sexual behaviors and relationships (see Coyne et al., 2019, for meta-analysis), less research has examined the influence of media on adolescents' sexual self-concepts (Deutsch et al., 2014). We focused on two feelings and two beliefs to reflect adolescent girls' sexual self-concept: sexual anxiety (i.e., tension/discomfort and negative judgments of one's sexual aspects in life; Snell, 1998), sexual self-esteem (i.e., affective reaction to subjective appraisals of sexual thoughts/feelings/behaviors; Doyle Zeanah & Schwarz, 1996), sexual self-efficacy (i.e., one's beliefs about their sexual abilities; Rosenthal et al., 1991), and enjoyment of sexualization (i.e., a belief whereby women desire to be admired for their sexual appeal/body parts/appearance; Liss et al., 2011).

Media effects on sexual self-concept

A relatively small body of literature has examined media effects on audiences' sexual self-concept, but these studies generally suggest that media consumption deflates college women's sexual self-concept (e.g., Aubrey, 2007; Seabrook et al., 2017; for exception, see Martino et al., 2005). We reviewed the literature of two constructs closely related to celebrity idolization – media fanship and celebrity worship. Media fanship, defined as regular, emotionally involved consumption of a popular narrative/text, was *negatively* related to adolescents' self-concept clarity (Dajches, 2022), suggesting that adolescents' fanship was related to *less* clearly defined self-concepts. Similarly, celebrity worship, defined as an extreme fascination with a famous person, was associated with higher anxiety in romantic relationships and poorer psychological well-being (Brooks, 2021). Like the studies on media consumption and the sexual self-concept (Aubrey, 2007; Seabrook et al., 2017), both media fanship and celebrity worship were related to *worse* outcomes for participants' identities and affect.

In the present study, we examine the associations between celebrity idolization and the sexual self-concept among U.S. adolescent girls. Since no research has studied celebrity idolization and the sexual self-concept, at least to our knowledge, we did not have a priori predictions about the direction of these relationships. Moreover, given that the existing research has utilized primarily heterosexual samples (e.g., Erickson & Dal Cin, 2018), we deemed it important to also include LGBQ+ girls in the present study. LGBQ+ celebrities mean a great deal to LGBQ+ adolescents. Bond (2018) found that LGBQ+ adolescents developed stronger parasocial relationships with LGBQ+ celebrities compared to heterosexual adolescents. Moreover, LGBQ+ celebrities fulfilled the role of confidants to LGBQ+ adolescents, especially among those who lacked real-life relationships with LGBQ+ individuals. Thus, just as with heterosexual participants, we expected that LGBQ+ adolescents would also understand their sexual self-concept through the depictions of LGBQ+ celebrities.

Method

Procedure

We recruited adolescent participants via a Qualtrics panel (e.g., a market research company that assists in recruiting participants). The Institutional Review Board at a large, public Southwestern university approved the study. Participants who were 18 years old indicated their agreement/consent, and for participants younger than 18, electronic consent was obtained from the parent and the child. Following consent, participants were provided with the following: "In the space provided, please indicate a celebrity who you find attractive. Although you may have multiple people you can think of, we'd like you to select only one." Participants then identified a celebrity, and their responses were pipe-texted into the celebrity idolization items.

Participants

Our sample consisted of 419 adolescent girls residing in the United States (13–18 years old, $M = 16.37$, $SD = 1.36$). Within this, 42.7% ($n = 179$) indicated their race as White, 17.2% ($n = 72$) as African American/Black, 14.1% ($n = 59$) as multi-ethnic/racial, 13.4% ($n = 56$) as Hispanic/Latinx, 7.6% ($n = 32$) as Asian/Asian American, 1.7% ($n = 7$) as American Indian/Native American/First Nation, 0.7% ($n = 3$) as South Asian, 0.5% ($n = 2$) as Middle Eastern, 0.2% ($n = 1$) selected "an ethnic/racial identity not listed," and 1.9% ($n = 8$) preferred not to answer. Concerning their relationship status, 66.6% (n = 279) identified as single, 20.8% (n = 39) were in a committed relationship, 9.3% (n = 39) were in a casual relationship, 1.9% (n = 8) selected "other," 0.7% (n = 3) were married, 0.5% (n = 2) were engaged, and 0.2% (n = 1) were separated.

For data analysis, we created a dichotomous variable for sexual identity grouping all adolescents who identified as LGBQ+ (i.e., bisexual, demisexual, gay, lesbian, pansexual, queer, questioning/unsure; 52.4%, n = 173) into one group and the heterosexual-identifying participants (47.6%, n = 181) into the other group. The 39 participants who preferred not to answer were not included in the analysis looking at sexual identity. Asexual participants would likely have less sexual or romantic interest in celebrity idols than the other participants. In total, 26 asexual participants were omitted from the analyses that included sexual identity.

Measures

To capture celebrity idolization, 16 items from Engle and Kasser's (2005) Celebrity Idolization Scale were used (α = .94). Sexual anxiety was measured using the Sexual Anxiety Subscale from the Sexual Self-Concept Questionnaire (MSSCQ; Snell, 1998; α = .89). Sexual self-esteem was assessed using the Sexual Self-Esteem Subscale from the Sexual Self-Concept Questionnaire (MSSCQ; Snell, 1998; α = .91). Sexual self-efficacy was measured using four items from Rostosky et al.'s (2008) Situational Self-Efficacy Scale and Resistive Self-Efficacy Scale (α = .79). Enjoyment of sexualization was measured using Liss et al.'s (2011) eight-item Enjoyment of Sexualization Scale (α = .86). Due to the sexual identity diversity within our sample, two similar versions of the scale were used; all of the items were the same, but the gender nouns were changed depending on participants' sexual identity. Plurisexual (i.e., LGBQ+ girls attracted to more than one gender) and heterosexual participants responded to the same version compared to monosexual participants (i.e., LGBQ+ girls attracted to one gender). Age and relationship status (coded as single or not single) were covariates in the analyses because they demonstrated moderate correlations with at least one of the dependent variables. For more details about the measures, see Measurement Appendix.

Results

Descriptive statistics

The selection of celebrity idols varied greatly across the sample. Harry Styles (4.3%; n = 18) and Zendaya (4.3%; n = 18), both film actors and songwriters, were the most frequently selected celebrities. Among hetero-sexual girls, film actors Tom Holland (7.2%; n = 13), Zac Efron (5.0%; n = 9), and Michael B. Jordan (5.0%; n = 9) were the most frequently selected. For LGBQ+ girls, Zendaya (9.0%; n = 18) was the most fre-quently selected, followed by Harry Styles (4.0%; n = 8), and then actors Tom Holland (2.5%; n = 5), Ian Somerhalder (2.5%; n = 5), and Matthew Gray Gubler (2.5%; n = 5). Table 7.1 displays the descriptive statistics and zero-order correlations between the main variables.

Main analyses

The adolescent girls' average celebrity idolization was just at the scale mid-point (M = 2.48, SD = 1.10) on the 1–5 scale. The highest scores were for the following two items: "I think [celebrity] is really hot" (M = 4.20, SD = 1.08) and "I am one of [celebrity's] biggest fans" (M = 3.47, SD = 1.24). None of the individual items significantly differed between heterosexual and LGBQ+ adolescents. The overall mean for celebrity idolization also did not differ between heterosexual (M = 2.46, SD = 1.12) and LGBQ+ girls (M = 2.40, SD = 1.04, t = −.54, p = .590).

We then conducted hierarchical regression models (HRMs), with age and relationship status entered in the first step and celebrity idolization entered in the second step, to examine the relationship between the adoles-cents' celebrity idolization and sexual self-concept. As displayed in Table 7.2, celebrity idolization was significantly related to each of the four dimensions of sexual self-concept. Celebrity idolization was *positively* related to sexual anxiety (β = .193, p < .001), sexual self-esteem (β = .125, p = .009), and enjoyment of sexualization (β = .133, p = .007) but was *negatively* related to sexual self-efficacy (β = −.101, p = .040).

To determine whether the results would hold up across sexual identity groups, we ran the HRMs again with sexual identity controlled. This anal-ysis restricted the sample to 353 participants who were categorized as either heterosexual or LGBQ+. For sexual anxiety, sexual esteem, and enjoyment of sexualization, celebrity idolization was related to each, as was found in the previous analyses. However, with sexual identity con-trolled, the association between celebrity idolization and sexual self-efficacy was reduced to non-significance (β = −.071, t = 1.33, p = .185).

We then examined the relations between celebrity idolization and the sexual self-concept variables by adolescent sexual identity (LGBQ+ or het-erosexual). As displayed in Table 7.3, many of the significant relationships reported above were found for heterosexual adolescent girls, such that celebrity idolization was positively related to sexual anxiety, sexual self-esteem, and enjoyment of sexualization. However, in contrast to our

TABLE 7.1 Zero-order correlations between the predictor, criterion, and demographic variables

Variables	M	SD	Min	Max	α	1.	2.	3.	4.	5.	6.	7.	8.
1. Celebrity Idolization	2.48	1.10	1.00	5.00	.94	1.00							
2. Sexual Anxiety	2.82	.98	1.00	5.00	.89	.20***	1.00						
3. Sexual Esteem	3.32	1.01	1.00	5.00	.91	.13*	.18***	1.00					
4. Sexual Efficacy	3.94	.99	1.00	5.00	.79	-.10+	-.09	.13*	1.00				
5. Enjoyment of Sexualization	4.10	1.30	1.00	7.00	.86	.14**	.16***	.31***	-.05	1.00			
6. LGBQ+	0.52	.50	0.00	1.00	-	-.03	.06	.09	.04	-.16**	1.00		
7. Age	16.36	1.37	13.00	18.00	-	.05	-.05	.15**	.09	.14**	-.13*	1.00	
8. RStatus	.67	.47	0.00	1.00	-	.03	.19***	-.19***	.00	.01	-.08	-.16***	1.00

Note: +p = .05; *p < .05; **p < .01; ***p < .001. LGBQ+ = LGBQ+ girls, RStatus = Relationship Status (Not single = 0, Single = 1).

TABLE 7.2 Hierarchical regression analyses testing relations between celebrity idolization and sexuality-related variables among all participants

	Sexual Anxiety	Sexual Esteem	Sexual Self-Efficacy	Enjoyment of Self-Sexualization
Step 1				
Single	.186***	−.201***	.016	.034
Age	−.024	.136*	.094	.141**
F	7.856***	9.523***	1.79	4.097*
Adj R^2	.031	.068	.004	.015
Step 2				
Single	.179***	−.207***	.019	.029
Age	−.034	.122*	.100	.134**
Celebrity Idolization	.193***	.163**	−.101*	.133**
F	10.924***	9.892***	2.63*	5.263**
Δ Adj. R^2	.037***	.024**	.010*	.015**

Note: Betas reported. $*p < .05$; $**p < .01$; $***p < .001$.

earlier inference, the relationship between celebrity idolization and sexual self-efficacy was not significant. For LGBQ+ adolescent girls, celebrity idolization was not related to any of the dimensions of sexual self-concept, except that sexual anxiety was almost positively related, but only at a level bordering significance ($p = .052$).

Discussion

According to the highest-rated celebrity idolization items, the celebrities that adolescent girls find attractive may function in two main ways: as romantic ("I think [celebrity] is really hot") and aspirational ("I am one of [celebrity's] biggest fans"). Furthermore, some of the lowest-rated items on the Celebrity Idolization Scale ("I have written to [celebrity]"; "I have lots of pictures, pinups, and posters for [celebrity]") suggest that celebrity idolization is less so happening via traditional "fan club" activities (e.g., writing letters, collecting pinups). Rather, modern celebrity idolization is likely occurring through social media. This includes following/liking/commenting on an idol's content or messaging other fans in online communities devoted to a particular idol (e.g., Discord, Reddit). Due to the rather exploratory nature of the present study, and the relative dearth of research on the topic, we used the original version of Engle and Kasser's (2005) Celebrity Idolization Scale to assess the state and utility of celebrity idolization among adolescent girls. However, we believe that an updated version of the scale should be used in future studies, especially considering the

TABLE 7.3 Hierarchical regression analyses testing relations between celebrity idolization and sexuality-related variables by sexual identity

	Heterosexual Participants				LGBQ+ Participants			
	Sexual Anxiety	Sexual Esteem	Sexual Self-Efficacy	ESS	Sexual Anxiety	Sexual Esteem	Sexual Self-Efficacy	ESS
Step 1								
Single	.239**	-.206**	-.024	.002	.172*	-.148*	.064	.038
Age	.033	.064	.014	.010	-.033	.205**	.165*	.262***
F	5.25**	4.49*	.080	.01	3.36*	8.25***	2.69	6.86**
Adj R^2	.045	.037	-.010	-.01	.023	.068	.017	.056
Step 2								
Single	.243***	-.203**	-.025	.007	.155*	-.156*	.074	.038
Age	.011	.033	.019	-.01	-.045	.199**	.173*	.261***
Celebrity Idolization	.242***	.189*	-.055	.249***	.138+	.065	-.086	.006
F	7.57***	5.36**	0.23	3.86*	3.55*	5.79***	2.29	4.55**
ΔAdj. R^2	.054***	.031*	.003	.057***	.014	.000	.002	-.05

Note: ESS = Enjoyment of Self-Sexualization. Betas reported. $+p = .05$; $*p < .05$; $**p < .01$; $***p < .001$.

interactive nature of celebrity idolization within the current media climate.

Although celebrity idolization may transpire in largely two disparate, but complementary ways, the primary idolization activities and attitudes captured via the Celebrity Idolization Scale (Engle & Kasser, 2005) were not significantly different when comparing heterosexual girls to LGBQ+ girls. This means that adolescent girls, regardless of sexual identity, engage in idolization for largely the same reasons – to express romantic/sexual feelings and to guide their aspirational goals. When examining all participants, controlling for sexual identity, the findings suggest that celebrity idols could be both a positive and, simultaneously, a negative influence on girls' sexual self-concepts. On a positive note, celebrity idolization was positively associated with sexual self-esteem. Celebrity idolization is often a one-way relationship, and perhaps girls feel safe and in control of managing that relationship. Celebrity idolization may also provide opportunities for retrospective imaginative involvement or further reflection/rumination on romantic/sexual feelings toward that celebrity, which may allow girls to envision their success in a romantic or sexual relationship (Slater et al., 2018).

On a negative note, celebrity idolization was also related to troubling components of the sexual self-concept for all participants. To start, celebrity idolization was connected to feelings of sexual anxiety perhaps because girls may feel that their celebrity idol is unattainable or out of reach. Adolescent girls may feel like they cannot match the ideal status of the celebrity they idolize, which may result in anxious feelings. Celebrity idolization was also positively associated with girls' enjoyment of sexualization, which means that having a celebrity idol was related to girls' *wanting* to be sexualized and evaluated based on their sexual appeal. Many of the celebrity idols identified within our sample could be regarded as sex objects, at least in the eyes of adolescent consumers (e.g., Harry Styles, Zac Efron). Therefore, we theorize that girls may adopt the same feelings of wanting to be sexualized in the same way that their celebrity idols invite sexualization.

Because adolescent girls' romantic and sexual feelings are riddled with contradictions (McRobbie, 1991), we should not be surprised that celebrity idols are related to both positive and negative aspects of their burgeoning sexuality. We suggest that parents and educators be cognizant of the subtle influences that can come from celebrity idols for girls' healthy sexual development and teach them about their sexual agency during their formative adolescent years. Parents could consider fostering spaces for shared dialogues about celebrities in relation to sexual knowledge and interests. Doing so has the potential to cultivate feelings of sexual self-esteem and promote a healthy curiosity related to girls' sexual self-concepts.

When examining celebrity idolization and sexual self-concept outcomes by sexual identity, differences emerged. For heterosexual girls, the results largely mirrored the findings for all participants, with the exception of sexual self-efficacy (which was reduced to non-significance). We conjecture that for heterosexual girls, celebrity idols likely provide a wealth of information that is related to heterosexual girls' understanding about matters related to sex and romance (e.g., gender roles, sexual interactions/expectations). It is important to note that the present study was cross-sectional, which limits the ability to make causal inferences. We suggest that future research should consider a longitudinal design to further explore the causal role of celebrity idols in the development of adolescent girls' sexual self-concept. Moreover, the present study is limited in that we asked participants to select a celebrity who they found "attractive." Future research would benefit from refining the definition of attraction to capture further nuance (e.g., social attraction or physical attraction).

For LGBQ+ adolescent girls, our results imply that celebrity idolization may not be a strong or particularly relevant source of sexual information. Celebrity idolization was only positively related to their sexual anxiety at a level bordering significance. That is, celebrity idolization, for the most part, was not significantly associated with elements of LGBQ+ adolescents' sexual self-concept. This could be partly due to the lack of "publicly out" LGBQ+ celebrity idols. In fact, within our sample, 76.8% ($n = 315$) of celebrity idols were coded as heterosexual/"publicly not out," compared to only 5.8% ($n = 24$) who were coded as LGBQ+/"publicly out." Due to the heteronormative media landscape (Van der Toorn et al., 2020), LGBQ+ girls may not see many LGBQ+ idols. Instead, LGBQ+ girls may look toward other resources to learn about their sexual self-concept. We suggest that LGBQ+ adolescents, in particular, may benefit from access to resources about LGBQ+ identities, relationships, and sexual interactions, including online resources and in-person resources such as an LGBQ+-friendly sex education curriculum.

Overall, developing and understanding one's sexual self-concept is an important developmental task (Rostosky et al., 2008), especially for adolescent girls. We conjecture that celebrity idols predominantly function as either targets for romantic/sexual development or as aspirational objects. Our results indicated that for heterosexual girls, idolization has positive and negative links to their sexual self-concept – perhaps suggesting that celebrities may be a promising avenue for media-related sex education programming. Yet, for LGBQ+ girls, idolization was only moderately linked to sexual anxiety, which indicates that there is more to understand as to how they come to develop and process their sexual self-concept beyond heteronormative celebrities.

References

Aubrey, J. S. (2007). Does television exposure influence college-aged women's sexual self-concept? *Media Psychology*, *10*(2), 157–181. https://doi.org/10.1080/15213260701375561

Bond, B. J. (2018). Parasocial relationships with media personae: Why they matter and how they differ among heterosexual, lesbian, gay, and bisexual adolescents. *Media Psychology*, *21*(3), 457–485. https://doi.org/10.1080/15213269.2017.1416295

Brooks, S. K. (2021). FANatics: Systematic literature review of factors associated with celebrity worship, and suggested directions for future research. *Current Psychology*, *40*(2), 864–886. https://doi.org/10.1007/s12144-018-9978-4

Caulfield, K. (2023, January 11). Bad Bunny's 'In Verano Sin Ti' is luminate's top album of 2022 in U.S. *Billboard*. https://www.billboard.com/music/chart-beat/2022-us-year-end-music-report-luminate-top-album-bad-bunny-un-verano-sin-ti-1235196736/

Coyne, S. M., Ward, L. M., Kroff, S. L., Davis, E. J., Holmgren, H. G., Jensen, A. C., ... & Essig, L. W. (2019). Contributions of mainstream sexual media exposure to sexual attitudes, perceived peer norms, and sexual behavior: A meta-analysis. *Journal of Adolescent Health*, *64*(4), 430–436. https://doi.org/10.1016/j.jadohealth.2018.11.016

Dajches, L. (2022). Finding the self through others: exploring fandom, identification, and self-concept clarity among U.S. adolescents. *Journal of Children and Media*, *16*(1), 107–116. https://doi.org/10.1080/17482798.2021.1922474

Deutsch, A. R., Hoffman, L., & Wilcox, B. L. (2014). Sexual self-concept: Testing a hypothetical model for men and women. *Journal of Sex Research*, *51*(8), 932–945. https://doi.org/10.1080/00224499.2013.805315

Doyle Zeanah, P., & Schwarz, J. C. (1996). Reliability and validity of the sexual self-esteem inventory for women. *Assessment*, *3*(1), 1–15. https://doi.org/10.1177/107319119600300101

Ehrenreich, B., Hess, E., & Jacobs, G. (1992). Beatlemania: Girls just want to have fun. In L. A. Lewis (Eds.) *The adoring audience: Fan culture and popular media* (pp. 84–106). Routledge.

Engle, Y., & Kasser, T. (2005). Why do adolescent girls idolize male celebrities? *Journal of Adolescent Research*, *20*(2), 263–283. https://doi.org/10.1177/0743558404273117

Erickson, S. E., & Dal Cin, S. (2018). Romantic parasocial attachments and the development of romantic scripts, schemas and beliefs among adolescents. *Media Psychology*, *21*(1), 111–136. https://doi.org/10.1080/15213269.2017.1305281

GLAAD Media. (2023). Where we are on TV 2022–2023. *GLAAD*. https://glaad.org/whereweareontv22/

Greene, A. L., & Adams-Price, C. (1990). Adolescent secondary attachments to celebrity figures. *Sex Roles*, *23*, 335–347. https://doi.org/10.1007/BF00289224

Jones, J. M. (2024, March 13). LGBTQ+ Identification in U.S. Now at 7.6% more than one in five Gen Z adults identify as LGBTQ+. *Gallup*. https://news.gallup.com/poll/611864/lgbtq-identification.aspx

Karniol, R. (2001). Adolescent females' idolization of male media stars as a transition into sexuality. *Sex Roles, 44*(1), 61–77. https://doi.org/10.1023/A:1011037900554

Khomami, N. (2022, September 30). 'A new kind of cross-media poly-talent: The cult of Harry Styles. *The Guardian.* https://www.theguardian.com/music/2022/sep/30/the-cult-of-harry-styles-dont-worry-darling

Kreager, D. A., Staff, J., Gauthier, R., Lefkowitz, E. S., & Feinberg, M. E. (2016). The double standard at sexual debut: Gender, sexual behavior and adolescent peer acceptance. *Sex Roles, 75*(7/8), 377–392. https://doi.org/10.1007/s11199-016-0618-x

Liss, M., Erchull, M. J., & Ramsey, L. R. (2011). Empowering or oppressing? Development and exploration of the Enjoyment of Sexualization Scale. *Personality and Social Psychology Bulletin, 37*(1), 55–68. https://doi.org/10.1177/0146167210386119

Martino, S. C., Collins, R. L., Kanouse, D. E., Elliott, M., & Berry, S. H. (2005). Social cognitive processes mediating the relationship between exposure to television's sexual content and adolescents' sexual behavior. *Journal of Personality and Social Psychology, 89*(6), 914–924. https://doi.org/10.1037/0022-3514.89.6.914

McRobbie, A. (1991). *Feminism and youth culture.* Macmillan.

Rosenthal, D., Moore, S., & Flyn, I. (1991). Adolescent self-efficacy, self-esteem, and sexual risk-taking. *Journal of Community & Applied Social Psychology, 1*(2), 77–88. https://doi.org/10.1002/casp.2450010203

Rosner, H. (2022, September 14). Harry Styles fans put on a show. *New Yorker.* https://www.newyorker.com/culture/photo-booth/harry-styles-fans-put-on-a-show

Rostosky, S. S., Dekhtyar, O., Cupp, P. K., & Anderman, E. M. (2008). Sexual self-concept and sexual self-efficacy in adolescents: A possible clue to promoting sexual health? *The Journal of Sex Research, 45*(3), 277–286. https://doi.org/10.1080/00224490802204480

Seabrook, R. C., Ward, L. M., Cortina, L. M., Giaccardi, S., & Lippman, J. R. (2017). Girl power or powerless girl? Television, sexual scripts, and sexual agency in sexually active young women. *Psychology of Women Quarterly, 41*(2), 240–253. https://doi.org/10.1177/0361684316677028

Slater, M. D., Ewoldsen, D. R., & Woods, K. W. (2018). Extending conceptualization and measurement of narrative engagement after-the-fact: Parasocial relationship and retrospective imaginative involvement. *Media Psychology, 21*(3), 329–351. https://doi.org/10.1080/15213269.2017.1328313

Snell, W. E. (1998). The multidimensional sexual self-concept questionnaire. In C. M. Davis, W. L. Yarber, R. Bauserman, G. Schreer, S. L. Davis (eds.), *Handbook of sexuality-related measures* (pp. 521–524). Sage.

Tukachinsky, R. (2010). Para-romantic love and para-friendships: Development and assessment of a multiple parasocial relationships scale. *American Journal of Media Psychology, 3*(1/2), 73–94.

Tukachinsky, R., & Dorros, S. M. (2018). Parasocial romantic relationships, romantic beliefs, and relationship outcomes in USA adolescents: Rehearsing love or setting oneself up to fail? *Journal of Children and Media, 12*(3), 329–345. https://doi.org/10.1080/17482798.2018.1463917

Van der Toorn, J., Pliskin, R., & Morgenroth, T. (2020). Not quite over the rainbow: The unrelenting and insidious nature of heteronormative ideology. *Current Opinion in Behavioral Sciences*, *34*, 160–165. https://doi.org/10.1016/j.cobeha.2020.03.001

Walker, S., Sanci, L., & Temple-Smith, M. (2013). Sexting: Young women's and men's views on its nature and origins. *Journal of Adolescent Health*, *52*(6), 697–701. https://doi.org/10.1016/j.jadohealth.2013.01.026

8

SECTION 1 COMMENTARY

Let's Talk About Mediated Sex: Using Media for
Sexual Identity Development

*Rebecca Ortiz, Jessica Fitts Willoughby, and
Stacey J.T. Hust*

Adolescents use media to explore and make sense of their gender and sexual identities during this important developmental time in their lives (e.g., Bates et al., 2019; Bond, 2018). The four chapters in this section summarized research that provided insight into how this can play out. The chapters examined how teens make sense of gendered and sexual representations they see in the media, and, specifically for LGBTQ teens, how they may use media to facilitate identity-based conversations with their parents, and, specifically for adolescent girls, how engagement with celebrities may impact how they see themselves sexually.

Hust et al. (Chapter 4) and L'Pree Corsbie-Massay (Chapter 5) found that while most of the teens in their research acknowledged that a person's gender identity and sexual orientation are not always outwardly apparent and sexuality exists on a spectrum, they still relied on stereotypical heteronormative frameworks to judge the content with which they engaged. In Hust et al.'s research, the teens commented on the physical attributes and mannerisms of the social media influencers when determining their gender identities, noting whether they presented as more stereotypically feminine or masculine and then correspondingly labeling them as female or male. When presented with the influencer's correct gender identity, different from what the teens presumed, they then used that information to determine the influencer's sexual orientation, labeling the influencers as gay or lesbian because they did not conform to stereotypical heteronormative gender expressions (e.g., a male beauty vlogger who presented as more stereotypically feminine).

DOI: 10.4324/9781032648880-10

Although these findings are not surprising, given that the teens relied on common cultural stereotypes and assumptions, it is interesting that the teens struggled regardless of their own gendered beliefs. The teens less likely to endorse gender role stereotypes (i.e., heterosexual scripts) were *not* necessarily less likely to misgender or misinterpret the sexuality of the social media influencers. Although the teens who endorsed heterosexual scripts did struggle to accept the influencer's correct gender identities, all the teens tapped into heteronormative standards and stereotypes when making their judgments, even the teens who noted that media representations of gender and sexuality had diversified in recent years.

The first-year communication college students in L'Pree Corsbie-Massay's research analyzed their favorite media content for presence or absence of sexuality representation. The media content favored by the students varied, but common themes emerged in how they judged the presence of sexuality. Many of the students coded their content as absent of sexuality while, at the same time, saying that it was comprised of heterosexual or straight characters. L'Pree Corsbie-Massay interpreted this to mean that the presence of heterosexuality is so normative and dominant that it does not compute as sexuality at all, unlike when non-heterosexual (e.g., lesbian, gay, bisexual, queer) characters or storylines were present. However, some of the students noted that when non-heterosexual/queer characters or storylines were present, they were often trivialized, serving as jokes, secondary characters, or tools to advance the main narrative, which many of the students identified as problematic. They expressed a desire for more nuanced, robust representations in the future and their hopeful involvement in making that happen as future creators and producers.

The teens in both Hust et al. and L'Pree's research used heteronormative frameworks to make sense of their media content, relying on assumptions about heterosexuality as the default and that feminine/masculine outward expression are indicative of the female/male gender binary and corresponding sexuality. However, teens in both studies also noted that these gender and sexual norms are rooted in historical context, such that they felt they were more progressive in their thinking than older generations who uphold more conservative and traditional norms. Although teens of today may, in fact, be generally more progressive in their beliefs and behaviors around gender and sexuality than previous generations, the teens here still struggle to totally break away from relying on these traditional frameworks to make sense of gender and sexuality. This echoes research from elsewhere. For example, results from interviews with 136 young people (aged 16–24) in the United Kingdom revealed that although the young people saw themselves as more accepting of gender diversity, they still experienced confusion and misunderstanding around the topic and may still hold greater comfort with stable and binary forms of gender (Allen et al., 2022). Despite this, as L'Pree Corsbie-Massay found, many young people are eager to put a critical lens on their media content and consider how they can contribute to creating media with more inclusive and diverse gender and sexuality representations.

The research presented in the other two chapters in this section further emphasized the need for more diverse media representations of sexuality and gender, with generational differences and tensions also highlighted in the research by Mares and Chen (Chapter 6). In their chapter, they presented results from reports by LGBTQ teens about their experiences co-viewing identity-related media content with their parents. As noted by the researchers, parental support can play a major role in the well-being of LGBTQ teens, and media representations of these identities can serve to open important parent–teen conversations. The researchers found that these conversations did not happen frequently, but when they did, they were generally more positive than negative. Teens noted that how their parents responded to an identity media portrayal, via such cues as facial expressions, comments, and willingness to watch the content, signaled to them whether they would receive support from the parent(s) in relation to their identity. But for these moments to happen, diverse representations must be more available and accessible for co-viewing.

Teens may also look to celebrities in the media to make sense of their identities, as highlighted in the research by Dajches and colleagues (Chapter 7). They found in their study with adolescent girls that heterosexual girls were just as likely as girls who identified as lesbian, gay, bisexual, or other sexual orientation or identity (LGBQ+) to engage in idolization of a celebrity they found attractive. However, when examining how this idolization relates to their sexual self-concepts (i.e., sexual anxiety, sexual self-efficacy, enjoyment of sexualization, and sexual esteem), it was only significant for heterosexual girls. The more heterosexual girls idolized their favorite celebrity, the more likely they were to report sexual anxiety, enjoyment of sexualization, and sexual esteem. This is both a concern and opportunity, such that it demonstrates that understanding more about how heterosexual girls look to celebrities for information about their sexuality could provide insight into how to ensure they develop healthy sexual self-concepts as a result and hopefully mitigate harmful effects.

But it also leaves unanswered questions about how this works for LGBQ+ girls, since they were just as likely to idolize a celebrity, but their idolization did not relate to their sexual self-concepts. Perhaps there are just not enough celebrities engaging in romantic and sexual representations that look like the kind these girls can relate to and therefore they do not impact them in the ways they do heterosexual girls. Heterosexuality is often the norm for many celebrity relationships and identities, and therefore finding relatable examples of sexuality among the celebrities LGBQ+ girls admire may be difficult.

The research presented across these four chapters highlights the significant role media can play in the development of teens' gender and sexual identities. Although today's teens are increasingly aware of the spectrum and complexity of gender and sexual identities, they may still resort to traditional heteronormative frameworks when interpreting media content. This is evident in how they misjudge influencers' gender identities and sexual orientations and perceive heterosexuality as the default sexual orientation. Even teens who see themselves as progressive in these areas can revert to these judgments. Heterosexuality as a sexuality remains dominant in most cultures, complicating the recognition and validation of LGBTQ+ identities by teens and the people they need to support them. More diverse and nuanced representations of gender and sexuality in the media may provide greater support for these teens, as relatable media personas may fill a gap in the lives of gender or sexual minority youths who do not have others in real life to which they can relate (Bond, 2018). The teens in some of the research presented in these chapters seemed to think so.

Research limitations must, however, be acknowledged. Most of the studies were conducted with convenience samples of youths in the United States, limiting the generalizability of the findings. Additionally, the cross-sectional nature of the research precludes any direct causal inferences. But these studies provide a snapshot of how media play a role in teens' lives as they develop their identities and underscore the necessity for teens to have access to media with positive and varied representations, thereby enabling teens to navigate their identities healthfully and confidently.

References

Allen, K., Cuthbert, K., Hall, J.J., Hines, S., & Elley, S. (2022). Trailblazing the gender revolution? Young people's understanding of gender diversity through generation and social change. *Journal of Youth Studies*, 25(5), 650–666. https://doi.org/10.1080/13676261.2021.1923674

Bates, A., Hobman, T., & Bell, B. T. (2019). "Let me do what I please with it ... Don't decide my identity for me": LGBTQ+ youth experiences of social media in narrative identity development. *Journal of Adolescent Research*, 35(1), 51–83. https://doi.org/10.1177/0743558419884700

Bond, B. J. (2018). Parasocial relationships with media personae: Why they matter and how they differ among heterosexual, lesbian, gay, and bisexual adolescents. *Media Psychology*, 21(3), 457–485. https://doi.org/10.1080/15213269.2017.1416295

SECTION 2

Princesses, Pornography, and Sexual Violence

Understanding the Impact of Teens' Experiences with Sexual Media Content

9

SECTION 2 INTRODUCTION

Princesses, Pornography, and Sexual Violence: Understanding the Impact of Teens' Experiences with Sexual Media Content

Stacey J.T. Hust

It is no longer surprising to read that young people have incorporated what they learn from the media into their romantic and sexual lives. In 2003, Collins and colleagues wrote about how television could be a "healthy sex educator," describing their results of a nationwide U.S. survey of teens who viewed and often remembered a message about condom efficacy in a popular television program. A couple of years later, Brown, Halpern and L'Engle (2005) published an article based on data obtained from more than 400 female adolescents in the U.S. state of North Carolina in which they stated that the "mass media may be serving as a kind of sexual super peer, especially for earlier maturing girls" (p. 420).

Since then, many more studies found effects of media on adolescent's sexual attitudes and behaviors in countries all around the world (e.g., Baams et al., 2015; Brown et al., 2006; Hust & Rodgers, 2018; Lin et al., 2020; Peter & Valkenburg, 2016; Ward, 2016). For example, Trekels et al. (2018) found that consumption of sexual media content was associated with girls' self-sexualization across a diverse sample from Austria, Belgium, Spain, and South Korea. An analysis of the longitudinal Taiwan Youth Project found that exposure to sexually explicit media was associated with the age of first sexual intercourse and unsafe sexual practices (Lin et al., 2020). Relatedly, in a review of 20 years of research from samples drawn around the world, Peter and Valkenburg (2016) described how adolescents' (ages 10–17) pornography use was associated with negative outcomes, such as gender stereotypical beliefs and sexual aggression, but that more scientifically robust research was needed to draw conclusions about causal effects. The chapters in this section extend what is currently known

DOI: 10.4324/9781032648880-12

about the influence of exposure to sexual media by considering the longer-term implications of such exposure and by questioning what happens when adolescents become engagers and producers, rather than merely consumers, of such content.

In 2012, Peggy Orenstein published the widely popular, *New York Times* best-selling book *Cinderella Ate My Daughter*, which resonated with readers who recognized and related to the princess phenomenon that occupied most girls' childhoods. Simultaneously, media scholars investigated the effects of watching Disney princess movies and engaging with princess culture on children. In Chapter 10, Ward and her colleagues explore whether recall of princess engagement and affinity during childhood is associated with young women's beliefs about their bodies, beliefs in self-sexualization, and courtship beliefs. Rather than considering simple exposure to princess movies, the authors account for active childhood engagement with mediated princess content, including dressing up and acting as princess characters. In recent years, Disney princesses have been shown to be more active and independent. Ward et al. consider whether a stronger childhood affinity toward specific groups of princesses (i.e., traditional princesses or adventurous princesses) is associated with adolescent girls' support of traditional courtship norms.

Our state-of-the-field research found close to 40% (38.8%, $n = 81$) of research published about teens, sex, and media focused on sexting (see Willoughby et al., Chapter 1). Given these results, it is perhaps not surprising that three of the four chapters in this section investigated the prevalence and effects of sexting on adolescents. However, these chapters offer unique contributions in their consideration of sexting and the effects of engaging in sexting on adolescents.

Much of the existing research on sexting has focused on older adolescents or young adults, but in Chapter 11, Van Ouytsel and colleagues question whether early adolescents (12–15 years old) in Belgium engage in image-based sexting, and whether boys and girls engage in these behaviors at different rates. The authors acknowledge the important role image-based sexting may play in teens' relationships, but they also recognize that some experiences with image-based sexts are non-consensual. The authors also consider early adolescents' experiences with image-based sexual abuse and adult online sexual solicitation.

Existing research has identified several factors associated with sexting behaviors, including normative beliefs, such that teens are more likely to engage in sexting if they perceive that their peers are also engaging in and accepting of such behavior (e.g., Maheux et al., 2020). In Chapter 12, Densley and colleagues extend this work by considering multiple antecedents to normative beliefs. They consider the effects of peer norms, measured by adolescents' perceptions of their close and distal peers' behaviors and beliefs, and the media, measured by exposure to pornography, on sexting behaviors.

Although most scholars recognize the potential harmful effects of adolescent engagement with sexting, Martínez-Bacaicoa and colleagues (in Chapter 13) extend this work to consider the use of digital technology to commit acts of sexual violence. The authors identify the prevalence of technology-facilitated sexual violence (TFSV), including (but not limited to) online gender-based violence, sextortion, and non-consensual sexting, among adolescents enrolled in schools in Spain. The authors use a longitudinal study (i.e., measurement over time) to determine changes in experiences with TFSV over time, to consider gender differences in the prevalence of TFSV victimization, and to test whether such experiences are associated with mental health outcomes such as anxiety and depression.

Overall, this section furthers our understanding of media effects by considering how engagement and content created by teens can impact teens' relationships and sexual attitudes and behaviors.

References

Baams, L., Overbeek, G., Dubas, J. S., Doornwaard, S. M., Rommes, E., & Van Aken, M. A. (2015). Perceived realism moderates the relation between sexualized media consumption and permissive sexual attitudes in Dutch adolescents. *Archives of Sexual Behavior, 44*, 743–754. https://doi.org/10.1007/s10508-014-0443-7

Brown, J. D., Halpern, C. T., & L'Engle, K. L. (2005). Mass media as a sexual super peer for early maturing girls. *Journal of Adolescent Health, 36*(5), 420–427. https://doi.org/10.1016/j.jadohealth.2004.06.003

Brown, J.D., L'Engle, K.L., Pardun, C.J., Guo, G., Kenneavy, K. & Jackson, C. (2006). Sexy media matter: Exposure to sexual content in music, movies, television and magazines predicts Black and White adolescents' sexual behavior. *Pediatrics, 117* (4), 1018–1027. https://doi.org/10.1542/peds.2005-1406

Collins, R., Elliott, M. N., Berry, S. H., Kanouse, D. E., & Hunter, S. B. (2003). Entertainment television as a healthy sex educator: The impact of condom-efficacy information in an episode of Friends. *Pediatrics, 112*(5), 1115–1121. https://doi.org/10.1542/peds.112.5.1115

Hust, S.J.T. & Rodgers, K.B. (2018) *Scripting adolescent romance: Adolescents talk about romantic relationships and media's sexual scripts.* Mediated Youth Series, Peter Lang Publishing.

Lin, W.H., Liu, C.H. & Yi, C.C. (2020). Exposure to sexually explicit media in early adolescence is related to risky sexual behavior in emerging adulthood. *PLOS ONE 15*(4), e0230242. https://doi.org/10.1371/journal.pone.0230242

Maheux, A. J., Evans, R., Widman, L., Nesi, J., Prinstein, M. J., & Choukas-Bradley, S. (2020). Popular peer norms and adolescent sexting behavior. *Journal of Adolescence, 78*, 62–66. https://doi.org/10.1016/j.adolescence.2019.12.002

Orenstein, P. (2012). *Cinderella ate my daughter*. Harper Books.

Peter, J., & Valkenburg, P. M. (2016). Adolescents and pornography: A review of 20 years of research. *The Journal of Sex Research*, 53(4–5), 509–531. https://doi.org/10.1080/00224499.2016.1143441

Trekels, J., Karsay, K., Eggermont, S., & Vandenbosch, L. (2018). How social and mass media relate to youth's self-sexualization: Taking a cross-national perspective on rewarded appearance ideals. *Journal of Youth and Adolescence*, 47(7), 1440–1455. https://doi.org/10.1007/s10964-018-0844-3

Ward, L. M. (2016). Media and sexualization: State of empirical research, 1995–2015. *Journal of Sex Research*, 53(4–5), 560–577. https://doi.org/10.1080/00224499.2016.1142496

10

WHAT BECOMES OF THE PRETTY PRINCESS?

Childhood Disney Princess Engagement and Affinity and Women's Appearance and Relationship Conceptions in Late Adolescence

L. Monique Ward, Jennifer Stevens Aubrey, Enrica Bridgewater, and Danielle Rosenscruggs

As icons of ideal femininity, Disney Princesses are often girls' first introductions to tales of love (Hefner et al., 2017). Yet scholars and educators have expressed concern that the emphasis on beauty and idealized romantic love in Disney Princess films may limit girls' conceptualizations of feminine roles and ideals (e.g., Orenstein, 2012). Moreover, girls not only *view* these Disney Princess portrayals but also engage with their ideals via toy play, pretend play, and dress-up. In this study, we explore downstream consequences of these experiences on girls' identity formation and beliefs about romantic relationships in late adolescence.

Disney Princess messages about appearance and romantic ideals

Although rules vary about what constitutes a Disney Princess film, they all feature a central female human character who may or may not be an actual princess and usually include a heterosexual romantic storyline. As of 2021, the Disney Princess universe encompasses 14 movies, from *Snow White and the Seven Dwarfs* (1937) to *Raya and the Last Dragon* (2021), excluding sequels and remakes. This lucrative franchise features numerous products, including clothing, games, toys, and décor, and is among the ten best-selling entertainment franchises, grossing $46.4 billion as of January 2021 (Romaine, 2021).

Content analyses of *early* Disney Princess films suggested that gender roles, especially for girls and women, were narrow and traditional. These princesses were passive, obedient, unusually quiet, and weak (Hefner et al.,

DOI: 10.4324/9781032648880-13

2017), and they were more likely than princes to display affection, fear, submission, sadness, and nurturing and grooming behaviors (England et al., 2011). However, over time, Disney Princesses became more well-rounded, determined, independent, and insistent on being true to themselves (Hine et al., 2018). In fact, in five of the recent Disney Princess films (*The Princess and the Frog, Tangled, Brave, Frozen,* and *Moana*), princesses exhibited more masculine characteristics, were equally represented in terms of rescue behaviors, and were less likely to get married than earlier Disney Princesses (Hine et al., 2018).

However, analyses indicate that both early *and* modern Disney Princess films emphasize beauty as an essential component of femininity (Hefner & Kretz, 2021) and value female characters for their appearance more than their intellect (Towbin et al., 2004). Moreover, the characters and accompanying merchandise epitomize unrealistic, thin ideals (Coyne et al., 2021). Content analyses also reveal idealized courtships that feature love at first sight, happily-ever-after storylines, and the quest for love as the ultimate pursuit (England et al., 2011; Hefner et al., 2017). The films promote a "relationship imperative," which suggests that the acquisitions of love and marriage are requirements for happiness (Hefner et al., 2017). In the first 12 Disney Princess movies, an average of 15.7 romantic ideals (e.g., love at first sight) and 11.8 challenges to these ideals were depicted per film. Idealized portrayals were typically rewarded with positive reactions, while challenges often elicited punishing and negative responses.

Disney Princesses and girls' self-beliefs

How does engagement with Disney Princess media and the idolization of Disney Princesses shape girls' beliefs about appearance and courtship? According to social cognitive theory (Bandura, 2001), children learn culturally appropriate behavior from direct teaching and from exposure to specific role models (e.g., parents, peers, media figures). Factors such as the attractiveness of the model, close connection with the model, and observed rewards or punishments influence the likelihood that the viewer will model her behavior. Disney Princesses may therefore be especially powerful models, given that they are attractive and prominent characters whose behaviors and courtship choices are often rewarded (e.g., living happily ever after). Moreover, by purchasing princess merchandise, parents encourage girls, explicitly or implicitly, to engage in play that highlights traditional femininity (Coyne et al., 2021).

Limited empirical evidence exists concerning the impact of Disney Princess media, with studies focusing mainly on young children and yielding mixed results. In one study, preschoolers' engagement with

Disney Princesses, defined as their frequency of viewing Disney Princess media, playing with Disney Princess toys, and identifying with princesses, was linked to higher levels of stereotypically feminine attributes, behaviors, and toy preferences, both initially and one year later (Coyne et al., 2016). Connections between Disney Princess engagement and children's body esteem were weaker and less consistent.

Experimental tests of the impact of a one-time Disney Princess exposure also yield inconsistent results. For example, girls wearing princess, neutral (e.g., pumpkin), or superhero costumes did *not* differ in their prosocial behaviors or perseverance task performance; thus, wearing princess costumes did not make girls behave more stereotypically "girly" (Coyne et al., 2021). Experiments investigating Disney Princess appearance messages have also produced weak effects (Bazzini et al., 2010; Hayes & Tantleff-Dunn, 2010). However, findings suggest that preschool girls do pay attention to princesses' beauty during play. In an observational study of Disney Princess play, preschool girls frequently called attention to and remarked on their appearance and invited others to do the same (Golden & Jacoby, 2018). Moreover, princess play often centered around costumes (e.g., tiaras) and unique body movements (e.g., twirling).

Although most studies have focused on young children, some research suggests downstream consequences of childhood Disney Princess engagement for young women's ideas about romantic relationships. When reflecting on the impact of Disney Princess culture on romantic love, most undergraduate women (ages 18–24) said that they distanced themselves from Disney Princess portrayals, considering them unrealistic, superficial, and simplistic; however, many desired selective components of idealized love, especially the "love conquers all" notion (Koontz et al., 2017). Moreover, childhood exposure to romantic ideals in 12 Disney Princess films had downstream consequences for one undergraduate sample (Hefner & Kretz, 2021). Although childhood exposure to romantic ideals in Disney Princess films did *not* predict students' current romantic beliefs, it did predict stronger belief that success in relationships is central to one's value as a person, especially among men, and greater endorsement of masculine courtship strategies. However, Hefner and Kretz (2021) focused solely on exposure, and richer results might be observed when Disney Princess engagement and affinity are assessed.

The current study

Although Disney Princesses are a critical aspect of many girls' childhood experiences, their status as feminine ideals may exact consequences for years to follow. We, therefore, focused on potential downstream consequences among late-adolescent women, who occupy a developmental period in which dating and sexual relationships are normative. We examined associations between older adolescents' recollections of childhood Disney Princess experiences and their current attitudes about appearance and courtship. Drawing on social cognitive theory, we focused on girls' engagement with Disney Princesses and affinity toward them (Bandura, 2001). We investigated the consequences of childhood Disney Princess engagement and affinity in three domains. We speculated that the heavy valuing of women's appearance and beauty in Disney Princess films and princess play would result in more negative body image *and* greater self-sexualization. Also, given Disney Princess culture's traditional courtship scripts, we expected that childhood engagement and affinity would predict stronger endorsement of traditional courtship beliefs.

Method

Participants

Undergraduate women (n = 647) aged 17–23 completed online surveys. Because we were interested in late adolescence, we eliminated those who were older than 21 (n = 24), yielding 623 participants for analysis (M = 18.74, SD = .91); 78.6% were 17–19. Participants could indicate multiple racial identities. In total, 429 (68.9%) selected White, 113 (18.1%) selected Asian/Asian-American/Pacific Islander (AAPI), 64 (10.3%) selected Latina, 43 (6.9%) selected Black/African-American, 18 (2.9%) selected Middle Eastern, five (0.8%) selected Native American/Alaskan, and 11 (1.8%) selected other. Additionally, 83.8% identified as exclusively heterosexual, 8.5% as predominantly heterosexual, 4.5% as bisexual, 0.8% as predominantly gay/lesbian, 0.2% as exclusively gay/lesbian, and 2.2% as not sure.

Procedure

Participants were recruited from participant pools at two U.S. universities, one in the Midwest (n = 458) and one in the Southwest (n = 165). Women enrolled in introductory classes were invited to complete a survey on the Qualtrics software platform for course credit. Study procedures were approved by the Institutional Review Boards at both universities.

Measures

Given our focus on Disney Princess engagement and affinity, we explain the Disney Princess variables in detail below. Because the criterion variables were based on established scales, we provide details about those variables in the Measurement Appendix.

Disney Princess engagement

This scale began with the following prompt:

> In the following questions, we are interested in whether and how much you engaged with Disney princesses in your media and play activities when you were growing up. We are interested in what you remember, as accurately as possible, about your Disney princess engagement when you were in early childhood, roughly 3–8 years old. Additionally, we ask you to limit your reflections to the following Disney Princesses when answering the following questions: Snow White (1937), Cinderella (1950), Aurora from *Sleeping Beauty* (1959), Ariel from *The Little Mermaid* (1989), Belle from *Beauty and the Beast* (1991), Jasmine from *Aladdin* (1992), Pocahontas (1995), and Mulan (1998).

Although *The Princess and the Frog* (2009), *Tangled* (2010), *Brave* (2012), *Frozen* (2013), and *Moana* (2016) were released at the time of data collection, they had not been released when participants were young children and so were excluded.

Six items, based on Coyne et al. (2016), assessed frequency of Disney Princess culture engagement. Participants used a six-point scale (0 = "never"; 5 = "very frequently") to indicate their frequency of viewing Disney Princess movies/shows; playing Disney Princess-related digital games; reading Disney Princess books; playing with Disney Princess toys; dressing up like Disney Princesses; and playing make-believe or role-playing games with Disney Princesses. Mean scores were computed across the items (α = .91); higher scores indicated heavier engagement.

Disney Princess affinity

Next, participants selected their favorite Disney Princess and answered 13 questions about their affinity for that princess. For this scale, we combined the five-item Wishful Identification Scale (Hoffner & Buchanan, 2005) with several items from the Parasocial Relationship Scale (Rubin & Perse, 1987), adapting items to Disney Princess language. For example, the original item "[He/she] is the sort of person I wanted to be like myself" became "[This princess] is the sort of person I wanted to be like myself." We subjected the 13 items to a Principal Components factor analysis with varimax rotation. The items loaded onto one factor, with loadings from

.50 to .76; this factor, labeled Princess Affinity, explained 44.1% of the variance ($\alpha = .89$).

Body beliefs

Body beliefs were assessed with three scales that focused on women's attendance to their body's appearance (OBCS-McKinley & Hyde, 1996), shame about their body matching the thin ideal (OBCS-McKinley & Hyde, 1996), and appreciation of body functionality (BAS-2, Tylka & Wood-Barcalow, 2015).

Self-sexualization

Self-sexualization was assessed with three scales that measured participants' enjoyment of a sexual appearance and sexual attention (ESS; Liss et al., 2011), participants' basing of their self-worth on their sexual appeal (SASW; Gordon & Ward, 2000), and frequency of self-sexualizing behavior (Smolak et al., 2014).

Courtship beliefs

Participants' support of traditional courtship norms was assessed using three scales. The Heterosexual Script Scale (Seabrook et al., 2016) examined endorsement of traditional sexual roles concerning commitment orientations, courtship strategies, and sexual modesty/prowess. The Romantic Beliefs Scale (Sprecher & Metts, 1989) examined the idealization of romantic relationships, including beliefs in one true love and love at first sight. The Romantic Relationships Subscale of the Conformity to Feminine Norms Inventory-45 (Parent & Moradi, 2010) assessed endorsement of a relationship imperative.

Covariates

We examined correlations between the nine criterion variables and multiple demographic variables and selected the following covariates that were significantly correlated with three or more outcomes: school (0 = Midwestern school; 1 = Southwestern school), mother's education, religiosity (mean of three items assessing religiosity, prayer frequency, and religious service attendance, each on a 1–5 scale), status as non-U.S. raised, identification as gay or bisexual, identification as Black, and identification as AAPI. We also controlled for relationship status for the courtship variables.

To isolate the contribution of Disney Princess engagement and affinity, beyond other forms of media use, we controlled for four media use variables. To assess consumption of popular TV programs with sexual content, participants used a 4-point scale (1 = Never; 4 = Quite a Bit) to indicate exposure to 50 programs, each rated as containing moderate to high levels of sexual content according to Common Sense Media. Mean scores were computed across the 50 items ($M = 1.64$, $SD = .30$; $\alpha = .83$). To indicate consumption of popular women's magazines known to feature relationship and sexual content, participants indicated how many issues per year (0–12) they read of 14 women's magazines (e.g., *Cosmopolitan, Elle*). We computed a mean score ($M = 0.61$, $SD = 1.05$; $\alpha = .90$). To indicate their music video consumption, participants reported how many hours (0–10+) they typically watch music videos on an average weekday, Saturday, and Sunday. A weekly music video sum was computed ($M = 3.72$, $SD = 9.26$). Finally, participants reported how many movies (0–10) they watch at the theater, on the computer/DVD, and on cable/streaming services during an average month. Responses were summed ($M = 7.1$, $SD = 4.3$).

Results

Descriptive statistics and inter-correlations for the main variables are provided in Table 10.1. Disney Princess engagement was high ($M = 4.21$, 1–6 scale), as was Disney Princess affinity ($M = 3.76$, 1–5 scale). Disney Princess engagement and affinity were correlated ($r = .54$, $p < .001$) but at a level that suggests that they are conceptually distinct. In total, 95.7% of participants selected a favorite Disney Princess, with Cinderella and Belle (*Beauty and the Beast*) receiving the most selections, and Snow White receiving the fewest (see Table 10.2).

Testing main research questions

We next examined whether Disney Princess affinity and engagement contribute to participants' appearance and courtship beliefs, beyond demographics and other media use. We ran nine multiple regression analyses, one for each criterion variable. We entered each demographic variable and general media variables on the first step, and the Disney Princess variables on the second step. Results are in Table 10.3. The first set of regressions tested whether Disney Princess engagement and affinity predicted women's body image. Some significant associations emerged as expected such that greater Disney Princess engagement was associated with higher levels of body surveillance. Likewise, stronger affinity for one's favorite

TABLE 10.1 Descriptives and zero-order correlations between main study variables

	PEngage	PAffinity	Surveill	Shame	Apprec	ESS	SSB	SASW	HSS	RomBel	Relate
PEngage	-----	.54***	.23***	.10*	-.02	.21***	.32***	.20***	.08	.05	.13**
PAffinity		-----	.24***	.19***	-.11**	.16***	.14***	.29***	.05	.06	.09*
Surveill			-----	.52***	-.50***	.34***	.22***	.48***	.18***	-.04	.15***
Shame				-----	-.61***	.18***	.10*	.40***	.17***	.06	.14***
Apprec					-----	.04	.17***	-.27***	-.09*	.06	-.02
ESS						-----	.50***	.39***	.58***	.21***	.22***
SSB							-----	.25***	-.12**	-.11**	-.06
SASW								-----	-.34***	-.17***	-.19***
HSS									-----	.27***	.35***
RomBel										-----	.37***
Relate											-----
Mean	4.21	3.76	4.16	3.21	3.66	4.00	3.91	1.67	2.80	4.34	3.25
SD	1.20	0.64	0.77	1.04	0.84	0.88	0.93	0.48	0.69	0.91	0.70

Note: *p < .05; **p < .01; ***p < .001. PEngage = Princess Engagement; PAffinity = Princess Affinity; Surveill = Body Surveillance; Apprec = Body Appreciation; ESS = Enjoyment of Sexualization Scale; SSB = Self-Sexualizing Behaviors; SASW = Sexual Appeal Self-Worth; HSS = Heterosexual Script Scale; RomBel = Romantic Beliefs; Relate = Romantic Relationships Subscale; SD = Standard Deviation.

TABLE 10.2 Favorite princess selected

Princess Type	N	Percentage
Group 1: Early Traditional Princesses		
Cinderella	125	20.1
Aurora (*Sleeping Beauty*)	48	7.7
Snow White	21	3.4
Group 2: Agentic but Sexualized Princesses		
Belle (*Beauty and the Beast*)	125	20.1
Ariel (*The Little Mermaid*)	87	14.0
Jasmine (*Aladdin*)	58	9.3
Group 3: Adventurer Princesses		
Mulan	87	14.0
Pocahontas	26	4.2
Other Responses		
None of these	26	4.2
Skipped	20	3.2

princess was associated with more body surveillance, greater body shame, and lower body appreciation. The second set of regressions tested whether Disney Princess engagement and affinity predicted self-sexualization. Findings confirmed our expectations such that greater Disney Princess engagement predicted greater enjoyment of sexualization and more frequent participation in self-sexualizing behaviors. Stronger affinity for one's favorite princess was associated with valuing oneself more for one's sexual appeal. The final set of regressions tested whether Disney Princess engagement and affinity were associated with courtship beliefs. Only one significant finding emerged, with stronger affinity for one's favorite princess predicting greater acceptance of idealized notions about romantic relationships.

Favoring a type of princess and traditional courtship norms

A stronger affinity for one's favorite princess predicted only the acceptance of romantic ideals, but we questioned whether favoring a type of princess was associated with weaker or stronger support of traditional courtship norms. Drawing on analyses outlining distinctions among the Disney Princesses (e.g., Reilly, 2016), we created three groups of princesses:

- Early Traditional (Group 1): Snow White, Cinderella, Aurora (*Sleeping Beauty*) – personify prettiness and passivity while awaiting rescue by a handsome prince

TABLE 10.3 Hierarchical regression analyses testing princess contributions above and beyond other contribution

	Body Image			Self-Sexualization			Courtship Beliefs		
	Surveill	Shame	Apprec	ESS	SSB	SASW	HSS	RomBel	Relate
Mother's Education	.01	-.02	.05	.08	.05	-.01	-.09*	-.08	-.01
Non-U.S. Raised	.04	-.00	-.01	-.01	.00	-.05	.02	-.01	-.06
Identify as Black	-.17***	-.19***	.13**	-.11*	-.04	-.18***	-.02	-.05	-.09*
Identify as AAPI	-.07	-.06	.02	-.13**	-.14***	.04	-.00	-.00	-.04
School	-.06	-.06	.07	-.05	.14**	.05	.12**	.13**	.07
Gay/Bisexual	-.02	.00	-.05	-.14***	-.09*	-.08	-.19***	-.13**	-.15***
Religiosity	.08	.04	.06	-.01	-.03	.06	.11**	.07	.07
In a Dating Relationship	---	---	---	---	---	---	-.10*	.23***	.12**
Sexy TV Programs	.09*	.01	.00	.20***	.12**	.08	-.00	-.05	-.07
Women's Magazines	-.03	-.01	.05	.08	.21***	.02	.09*	.08	.09*
Music Videos/Week	-.05	.00	.00	.04	-.02	.01	.12**	.08	-.00
Movies/Month	.01	.08	-.05	-.06	.03	-.08	-.01	.02	-.04
Princess Engagement	.13**	-.03	.05	.13**	.24***	.04	.02	-.02	.07
Princess Affinity	.13**	.18***	-.11*	.05	.01	.25***	.09	.11*	.06
Step 1: Demos and Media Adj. R^2	.057	.032	.018	.127	.184	.053	.100	.099	.052
Step 2: Princess Media Adj. R^2	.101	.054	.022	.149	.240	.119	.107	.106	.061
Change in Adj. R^2	+.044***	+.022***	+.004	+.022***	+.056***	+.066***	+.007	+.007*	+.009*
Final Equation F	5.95***	3.51***	2.01*	8.69***	14.86***	6.85***	5.84***	5.81***	3.62***

Note: $*p < .05$; $**p < .01$; $***p < .001$. Betas from final step reported. Surveill = Body Surveillance; Appc = Body Appreciation; ESS = Enjoyment of Sexualization; SSB = Self-Sexualizing Behaviors; SASW = Sexual Appeal Self-Worth; HSS = Heterosexual Script Scale; RomBel = Romantic Beliefs; Relate = Romantic Relationships subscale.

TABLE 10.4 Analyses of variance testing differences in courtship beliefs based on favorite princess

	Early Traditional Group 1	Agentic but Sexualized Group 2	Adventurer Group 3	F
Heterosexual Script (HSS)	2.94$_a$	2.74$_b$	2.65$_b$	8.259***
Romantic Beliefs (RomBel)	4.50$_a$	4.28$_b$	4.14$_b$	6.466**
Support Relationship Imperative (Relate)	3.36$_a$	3.27$_a$	3.01$_b$	8.947***

Note: Differing subscripts reflect a statistically significant difference, via post-hoc Scheffé tests. $**p < .01$; $***p < .001$.

- Agentic but Sexualized (Group 2): Ariel, Belle, Jasmine – more agentic but also more sexualized (Belle is an outlier as she was far more agentic than she was sexualized)
- Adventurer (Group 3): Pocahontas, Mulan – fight for their group/ nation; less central romantic storyline

We then examined whether means for the three courtship variables differed based on which princess was selected as the favorite. As reported in Table 10.4, participants' endorsement of courtship norms did indeed differ significantly based on their favored princess. Respondents who favored a Disney Princess in Group 1 expressed greater support of the heterosexual script and romantic ideals than respondents who favored a Disney Princess in Group 2 or Group 3. Also, respondents in Groups 1 and 2 were more supportive of a relationship imperative than those in Group 3. Overall, young women who selected Pocahontas or Mulan as their favorite princess were significantly less invested in traditional courtship norms.

Discussion

The Disney Princess line is not only a lucrative, salient, and popular media franchise, but Disney Princesses also symbolize ideal courtship and femininity for many girls. Scholars have expressed concern that the idealized portrayals of courtship and overemphasis on women's beauty and appearance may encourage body image concerns, preoccupation with one's sexual appeal, and unrealistic and idealized courtship beliefs (e.g., Orenstein, 2012). Although these ideas have been studied among preschoolers (e.g., Coyne et al., 2016), less attention has focused on downstream consequences into late adolescence. We therefore addressed that angle here.

Our most consistent findings related to body image and self-sexualization. The emphasis on beauty in Disney Princess culture likely reinforces the notion that women's main value comes from their appearance, a schema that is established through early gender socialization and reinforced through the Disney Princess idolization. In childhood, these ideas likely manifest in seemingly innocent play (Golden & Jacoby, 2018). However, internalizing messages that characterize attractiveness as one's greatest asset may later contribute to body insecurities and a tendency to self-sexualize in adolescent girls. Thus, Disney Princesses might be one avenue by which girls are groomed to value being objectified. This early grooming can have lasting consequences for young women's sexual health, as self-sexualization predicts lower levels of sexual satisfaction, sexual esteem, and sexual assertiveness, and greater sexual monitoring and engagement in sexual risk behaviors (Ward et al., 2023). These findings suggest that women's ability to advocate for their needs and to derive pleasure from their sexual encounters can be compromised when they give greater attention to how their body looks than how it feels.

In terms of courtship beliefs, young women who favored a more modern Disney Princess (i.e., Pocahontas, Mulan) were significantly less invested in traditional courtship norms. A likely explanation for this distinction is that neither Pocahontas nor Mulan had a "happily ever after" romantic resolution (Reilly, 2016). For example, Pocahontas chose to stay with her family instead of following John Smith to England, and Mulan was less concerned with marriage and was more motivated by family duty and honor. Thus, participants who idolize those princesses were probably not as concerned with romance or courtship when they were younger and perhaps are less driven by romantic pursuits in late adolescence. It is also noteworthy that portrayals of princesses in Disney Princess films have evolved since 2009 such that modern Disney Princesses are more independent and self-sufficient. Teen girls who idolize princesses such as Elsa (*Frozen*) or Merida (*Brave*) may also be less concerned with traditional courtship beliefs, like those who identified with Pocahontas and Mulan.

Unexpectedly, Disney Princess affinity and engagement produced only one significant association with young women's courtship beliefs. A stronger affinity for one's favorite princess was associated with greater support of romantic ideals (e.g., love at first sight). This finding contrasts with Hefner and Kretz's (2021) study that found no relationship between Disney Princess film exposure and romantic beliefs. The authors suggested that viewing alone might not explain the connections with later romantic beliefs, and our analyses suggest that Disney Princess affinity, which reflects an ongoing imaginative involvement with the character, could be more critical to viewers' romantic beliefs than discrete exposure. Still, we must recognize that the five other tests of this hypothesis did not support our expectation that Disney Princess engagement and affinity would be correlated with traditional courtship beliefs. Perhaps the influences of Disney Princesses are limited in late adolescence, as young women distance themselves from their unrealistic romantic models (Koontz et al., 2017).

These findings are qualified by several limitations. Employing retrospective self-reports of Disney Princess engagement and affinity introduces recall biases into assessments. However, we reason that Disney Princesses were likely salient and memorable childhood role models. Additionally, the cross-sectional design prevents us from making causal conclusions. Longitudinal studies are needed to further assess the downstream consequences of Disney Princess engagement and affinity. Finally, our somewhat racially homogenous sample limits generalizability to broader populations.

Despite these limitations, our findings suggest that childhood Disney Princess engagement and affinity are associated with young women's negative body image, increased self-sexualization, and a stronger belief in romantic ideals. In particular, the extent to which girls engage with and idolize Disney Princesses appears to emphasize rigid feminine norms to which young women try to adhere to, even in late adolescence. Additionally, preferring earlier and more traditional princesses, such as Cinderella, appears to reflect greater support of romantic ideals and traditional sexual roles.

References

Bandura, A. (2001). Social cognitive theory of mass communication. *Media Psychology*, 3(3), 265–299. https://doi.org/10.1207/S1532785XM EP0303_03

Bazzini, D., Curtin, L., Joslin, S., Regan, S., & Martz, D. (2010). Do animated Disney characters portray and promote the beauty-goodness stereotype? *Journal of Applied Social Psychology*, 40, 2687–2709. https://doi.org/10.1111/j.1559-1816.2010.00676.x

Coyne, S., Linder, J., Rasmussen, E., Nelson, D., & Birkbeck, V. (2016). Pretty as a princess: Longitudinal effects of engagement with Disney princesses on gender stereotypes, body esteem, and prosocial behavior in children. *Child Development*, 87(6), 1909–1925. https://doi.org/10.1111/cdev.12569

Coyne, S., Rogers, A., Shawcroft, J., & Hurst, J. (2021). Dressing up with Disney and make-believe with Marvel: The impact of gendered costumes on gender typing, prosocial behavior, and perseverance during early childhood. *Sex Roles*, 85(5–6), 301–312. https://doi.org/10.1007/s11199-020-01217-y

England, D., Descartes, L., & Collier-Meek (2011). Gender role portrayal and the Disney princesses. *Sex Roles*, 64(7–8), 555–567. https://doi.org/10.1007/s11199-011-9930-7

Golden, J. C., & Jacoby, J. W. (2018). Playing princess: Preschool girls' interpretations of gender stereotypes in Disney princess media. *Sex Roles*, 79(5–6), 299–313. https://doi.org/10.1007/ s11199-017-0773-8

Gordon, M. K., & Ward, L. M. (2000, March). I'm beautiful, therefore I'm worthy: Assessing associations between media use and adolescents' self-worth. Paper presented at the *Biennial Meeting of the Society for Research on Adolescence*, Chicago, IL.

Hayes, S., & Tantleff-Dunn, S. (2010). Am I too fat to be a princess? Examining the effects of popular children's media on young girls' body image. *British Journal of Developmental Psychology, 28*(2), 413–426. https://doi.org/10.1348/02615 1009X424240

Hefner, V., Firchau, R., Norton, K., & Shevel, G. (2017). Happily ever after? A content analysis of romantic ideals in Disney princess films. *Communication Studies, 68*(5), 511–532. https://doi.org/10.1080/10510974.2017.1365092

Hefner, V., & Kretz, V. (2021). Does the glass slipper fit? Disney Princess films and relationship beliefs and attitudes. *Journal of Media Psychology, 33*(3), 125–133. https://doi.org/10.1027/18641105/a000290

Hine, B., England, D., Lopreore, K., Horgan, E. S., & Hartwell, L. (2018). The rise of the androgynous princess: Examining representations of gender in prince and princess characters of Disney movies released 2009–2016. *Social Sciences, 7*(245). https://doi.org/10.3390/socsci7120245

Hoffner, C., & Buchanan, M. (2005). Young adults' wishful identification with television characters: The role of perceived similarity and character attributes. *Media Psychology, 7*(4), 325–351. https://doi.org/10.1207/S1532785XMEP0 704_2

Koontz, A., Norman, L., & Okorie, S. (2017). Realistic love: Contemporary college women's negotiations of princess culture and the "reality" of romantic relationships. *Journal of Social and Personal Relationships, 36*(2), 535–555. https://doi.org/10.1177/0265407517735694

Liss, M., Erchull, M. J., & Ramsey, L. R. (2011). Empowering or oppressing? Development and exploration of the Enjoyment of Sexualization scale. *Personality and Social Psychology Bulletin, 37*(1), 55–68. https://doi.org/10.1177/0146167210386119

McKinley, N. M., & Hyde, J. S. (1996). The objectified body consciousness scale: Development and validation. *Psychology of Women Quarterly, 20*(2), 181–215. https://doi.org/10.1111/j.1471-6402.1996.tb00467.x

Orenstein, P. (2012). *Cinderella ate my daughter*. Harper Books.

Parent, M., & Moradi, B. (2010). Confirmatory factor analysis of the Conformity to Feminine Norms Inventory and development of an abbreviated version: The CFNI-45. *Psychology of Women Quarterly, 34*(1), 97–109. https://doi.org/10.1 111/j.1471-6402.2009.01545.

Reilly, C. (2016). An encouraging evolution among Disney princesses? A critical feminist analysis. *Counterpoints, 477*, 51–63. https://www.jstor.org/stable/45157186

Romaine, J. (2021, October 7). *The top 10 media franchises*. The Hill. https://thehill.com/changingamerica/enrichment/arts-culture/575813-the-top10media franchises/.

Rubin, A., & Perse, E. (1987). Audience activity and soap opera involvement: A uses and effects investigation. *Human Communication Research, 14*(2), 246–268. https://doi.org/10.1111/j.1468-2958.1987.tb00129.x

Seabrook, R., Ward, L. M., Reed, L., Manago, A., Giaccardi, S., & Lippman, J. (2016). Our scripted sexuality: The development and validation of a measure of the heterosexual script and its relation to television consumption. *Emerging Adulthood, 4(5)*, 338–355. https://doi.org/10.1177/2167696815623686

Smolak, L., Murnen, S. K., & Myers, T. A. (2014). Sexualizing the self: What college women and men think about and do to be "sexy." *Psychology of Women Quarterly, 38*(3), 379–397. https://doi.org/10.1177/0361684314524168

Sprecher, S., & Metts, S. (1989). Development of the 'Romantic Beliefs Scale' and examination of the effects of gender and gender-role orientation. *Journal of Social and Personal Relationships, 6*(4), 387–411. https://doi.org/10.1177/0265407589064001

Towbin, M., Haddock, S., Zimmerman, T. S., Lund, L. K., & Tanner, L. R. (2004). Images of gender, race, age, and sexual orientation in Disney feature-length animated films. *Journal of Feminist Family Therapy, 15*(4), 19–44. https://doi.org/10.1300/J086v15n04_02

Tylka, T., & Wood-Barcalow, N. (2015). The Body Appreciation Scale-2: Item refinement and psychometric evaluation. *Body Image, 12*, 53–67. https://doi.org/10.1016/j.bodyim.2014.09.006

Ward, L. M., Daniels, E., Zurbriggen, E., & Rosenscruggs, D. (2023). The nature, sources, and consequences of sexual objectification. *Nature Reviews Psychology, 2*(8), 496–513. https://doi.org/10.1038/s-44159-023-00192-x

11

IMAGE-BASED SEXTING AND SEXUAL ABUSE EXPERIENCES AMONG EARLY ADOLESCENTS

Joris Van Ouytsel, Chelly Maes, and Laura Vandenbosch

Digital media provide adolescents with ways to engage in sexual communication with others, such as via sexting. Sexting is defined in various ways by researchers; some define sexting as the sending or receiving of self-created sexually explicit text messages, images, and/or videos via the internet or mobile phone, such as via mobile phone text message or direct message on an internet application or website (Van Ouytsel et al., 2021). Others prefer a narrower definition of sexting, focused only on self-made sexually explicit images or videos (Van Ouytsel et al., 2021). A common denominator across definitions of sexting is the self-made aspect of the content, such that sexting is distinct from other forms of online sexual behavior and communication, such as the exchange of commercial pornography (i.e., pornography made by others for profit motives) (Vanden Abeele et al., 2014).

Depending on the definition used (i.e., focused on textual and/or visual content), researchers may obtain different results concerning the prevalence, motivations, and consequences of sexting by adolescents. For example, adolescents are more likely to engage in text-based forms of sexting compared to image-based sexting, which means that combining text-based forms of sexting and image-based forms of sexting in one measurement could lead to inflated prevalence rates (Maes & Vandenbosch, 2022). Furthermore, sexually explicit text-based sexting may have different outcomes compared to visual forms of sexting (Courtice & Shaughnessy, 2021). When a sexually explicit image-based message is distributed beyond its intended audience, it can lead to enduring psychological and social consequences (Bindesbøl Holm Johansen et al., 2019). In this chapter, we,

DOI: 10.4324/9781032648880-14

therefore, examine and define sexting as the sending of self-made sexually explicit pictures through the internet or the mobile phone to others as a narrow definition allows us to better understand this risky behavior that may have serious psychosocial consequences for youth (Courtice & Shaughnessy, 2021).

Why do adolescents engage in sexting?

For some, sexting is part of their relational and sexuality development (Choi et al., 2019; Van Ouytsel et al., 2021). A meta-analysis of sexting studies worldwide found that prevalence rates of sexting increase as adolescents mature, and adolescent boys and girls are sending sexts at the same rate (Madigan et al., 2018). Many adolescents initiate sexting in their first romantic relationships, and for some, engagement in sexting may be a less intrusive way to experiment with their sexuality compared to offline sexual contact (Choi et al., 2019). It can also be a way to signal to their partners that they are ready to take the relationship to the next level (Huntington & Rhoades, 2021). Youth who engage in sexting are more likely to be involved in offline sexual behaviors than their peers (Choi et al., 2019).

Peer pressure from adolescents' social network can also steer their engagement in sexting (Walrave et al., 2015). During adolescence, the opinions of peers begin to exert a greater influence (Walrave et al., 2015). Studies find that when adolescents perceive that their friends approve of sexting, they are more likely to engage in the behavior (Walrave et al., 2015). Boys may feel pressured by peers to engage in sexting as a sign of maturity, while girls in heterosexual relationships often experience pressure from romantic partners and fear relationship consequences if they refuse (e.g., their partner may end the relationship or lose interest) (Maes & Vandenbosch, 2022; Ringrose et al., 2013). Those who engage in sexting under partner pressure tend to send more explicit messages (e.g., depictions of sexual acts) (Maes & Vandenbosch, 2022).

Adolescents primarily engage in sexting within romantic relationships to maintain intimacy (Van Ouytsel et al., 2021). Given that adolescents typically cannot reside with their romantic partners, sexting can become a way to sustain intimacy within their long-distance relationships or during holidays, weekends, or school vacations (Van Ouytsel et al., 2021). Despite these relational motivations, research suggests sexting does not necessarily enhance relationship satisfaction (Van Ouytsel et al., 2019). Even more, for some adolescents sexting could be indicative of negative relational experiences, such as verbal conflict with their romantic partner (Huntington & Rhoades, 2021).

Image-based sexual abuse

Sexting is problematic and constitutes a form of image-based abuse when there is no mutual consent between the adolescents, such as when one is pressured to engage in sexting or when images are distributed without consent (Ringrose et al., 2022). Sometimes adolescents may also receive unwanted sexts, such as when someone sends a sexual image to another person without being asked to do so (Ringrose et al., 2022). Unwanted sexts can come from adults, friends, or partners. Sometimes boys may send an unwanted sext as a way to put pressure on their partner to send a message themselves; in other cases, they can be sent to sexually harass the victims (Ringrose et al., 2022).

The most well-known risk of sexting is that of non-consensual forwarding, such that sexual images are forwarded to others or published without permission of the original creator. The perpetrators may not always forward the images directly but may also share them on their mobile phone screens to others in person. In some cases, the images are spread when a romantic relationship ends (Bindesbøl Holm Johansen et al., 2019), or images might be forwarded to enhance one's popularity in the peer group, to gossip (Casas et al., 2019), or to showcase sexual maturity (Ringrose et al., 2013). Some youths may downplay the act of forwarding sexts as a "joke," which reduces the likelihood of recognizing the behavior as abusive (Van Ouytsel et al., 2021). Oftentimes, the victim whose images are distributed is blamed for the unauthorized forwarding of their messages, which can then contribute to a victim's hesitancy to seek help (Maes et al., 2023). Victim-blaming beliefs are even associated with a higher willingness to engage in the non-consensual forwarding of sexts (Maes et al., 2023).

Sexting images can be used to extort the victims (i.e., sextortion) (Paat & Markham, 2021), where perpetrators threaten to release the images unless victims comply with their requests. Perpetrators may obtain images through shared sexts or hacking the victim's computer or mobile phone (Paat & Markham, 2021). Often, perpetrators are known to the victim (e.g., [ex-]partners), though they can also be unknown (e.g., stalkers or criminals located abroad) (Patchin & Hinduja, 2020). Some use deep fakes and artificial-intelligence-generated images, posing a growing concern.

Victims of sextortion suffer long-term psychological consequences, including bullying, trust issues, reputational damage, anxiety, depression, a deteriorated self-esteem, and even indicators of posttraumatic stress syndrome (Pampati et al., 2020). Victims may avoid school due to shame, and removal of online images is difficult, with victims often living with the fear that images resurface (Bindesbøl Holm Johansen et al., 2019). Even though consequences for victims are severe, witnesses rarely intervene (Van Ouytsel et al., 2021).

The present study

With this study, we aim to map the prevalence of image-based sexting and sexual abuse experiences among a sample of early adolescents (12–15 years old) in Belgium. Early adolescents are a vulnerable age group for the risks associated with sexting, as they are often less mature than older adolescents when it comes to navigating situations such as peer pressure to engage in sexting (Madigan et al., 2018). Most studies on sexting focus on young adults and older adolescents, so our study addresses the need for literature on sexting to focus on younger and vulnerable age groups (Van Ouytsel et al., 2021). Although both boys and girls engage equally in sending sexts, certain aspects of sexting, such as forwarding explicit messages and engaging in sexting under pressure, are gendered. Therefore, our study seeks to focus on sex differences related to various sexting variables.

Although our study was conducted in Dutch-speaking provinces of Belgium and questions can be raised regarding local cultural differences, prior research found very little difference in the frequency of teenagers' sexting across countries (Madigan et al., 2018). Yet, some differences exist in offline sexual behaviors. For example, youths in the Netherlands, a neighboring country from Belgium, were found to engage in sexual activities at a later age and were more likely to discuss sexual health with their parents than their U.S. counterparts (van de Bongardt et al., 2014).

Method

Sample and procedures

In the Spring of 2019, the data for this study was collected as part of the second wave of a larger survey on adolescent risk behaviors and digital media use in Belgium. Participants filled in anonymous surveys in schools. Although efforts were made to reach a diverse sample of adolescents, we employed a convenience sample of participants. The sample consisted of 2,644 adolescents aged 12–15 ($M = 13.45$, $SD = .90$), which may not fully represent the broader adolescent population. The study was cross-sectional, which means that it was conducted at one point in time and that we were not able to track the behaviors of the participants over a longer time. Ethical approval was obtained from the University of Antwerp's ethical committee, and the study was supported by the Research Foundation Flanders (12J8719N) and Research Fund of the University of Antwerp (BOF Klein Project – FFB180048). Participants were given the option to skip questions. Before conducting the survey, permission was secured from school administration, and passive parental consent and adolescent assent were obtained. To mitigate self-report bias (e.g., some participants might have been reluctant to report their sexting behaviors), anonymity was stressed to the participants, we arranged the classrooms in a test-like setting, and participants were asked to return surveys in sealed envelopes.

Measures

Image-based sexting

First, adolescents were provided with our definition of sexting (i.e., sending and receiving self-made sexually explicit pictures through the internet or the mobile phone). We then asked if they had ever sent, received, or asked someone to send an image-based sext based upon this definition. The items were adapted from previous literature on sexting (Van Ouytsel et al., 2014; Van Ouytsel et al., 2019). We measured the items on a Likert-type scale ranging from 1 = *never* to 5 = *very often*. Because on average, the behaviors did not occur very often (e.g., sending of image-based sexts had a Mean (M) = 1.15; SD = .51), we recoded them into 1 = *did not experience the behavior*, and 2 = *experienced the behavior*.

Image-based sexual abuse

Adolescents were then asked if they had even been pressured to send a sexually explicit image of themselves or if they had engaged in non-consensual forwarding of an image-based sext. These two items were adapted from the "Questionnaire for Online Sexual Solicitation and Interaction of Minors with Adults" (Gámez-Guadix et al., 2018). We measured the items on a Likert-type scale ranging from 1 = *never* to 5 = *very often*. In a separate 4-item Likert scale, the adolescents were also asked about adult online sexual solicitation experiences in the year prior to the survey (i.e., whether an adult had ever asked them to send an image-based sext or had sent them one). Participants were asked to recall behaviors with individuals they perceived to be older than 18 years. Because on average, the behaviors in both scales did not occur very often (e.g., the item on being asked to send an image-based sext had M = 1.14; SD = .47), we recoded them into 1 = *did not experience the behavior* and 2 = *experienced the behavior*.

Independent variables

We asked participants to indicate their age, frequency of internet use, and their sex. Frequency of internet use was included as an independent variable in data analysis, as previous studies found that frequency of internet use was associated with engagement in sexting behavior (Mitchell et al., 2012). Participants were asked how frequently they used the internet ranging on a five-point Likert-type scale from 1 = *less than once a week* to 5 = *almost constantly* (M = 4.28; SD = .75) (Pew Research Center, 2018).

Sex was measured as a binary variable (male/female). In our sample, 1,124 participants (42.5%) were male, 1,466 participants were female (55.4%), and 54 participants (2.0%) did not provide a response. The latter group was excluded from the analysis. We acknowledge that measuring sex as a binary variable is a serious limitation of our study and that, moving forward, researchers should incorporate more diverse measures of gender that capture a variety of gender identities in their sexting studies. For further details about the measurements used in this chapter, please see the Measurement Appendix.

Data analysis

We used SPSS version 27.0 (IBM Corp, Armonk, NY). We conducted a series of multiple logistic regression analyses, each focusing on a different sexting behavior included in our research. Distinct models were utilized for each outcome variable. The sexting behaviors were used as dependent variables. We entered sex, age, and frequency of internet use as independent variables. Missing values on the variables were excluded from the analyses using listwise deletion.

Results

As shown in Table 11.1, 9.6% of adolescents had sent an image-based sext, and 34.2% had received one. For image-based sexual abuse, 10.9% of the participants had been pressured to send a sext of themselves, and 6.7% had engaged in the non-consensual forwarding of sexts. For online adult sexual solicitation, 9.6% of adolescents had experiences with an adult requesting that they send an image-based sext, and 15.5% received an image-based sext from an adult.

As shown in Tables 11.2 and 11.3, being older and greater internet use were significantly associated with all image-based sexting and sexual abuse behaviors. Thus, adolescents who are older and youth who are more frequently online are more likely to engage in image-based sexting and experience image-based sexual abuse.

As for differences by sex, boys were more likely than girls to have non-consensually forwarded an image-based sext (5.3% for girls vs. 8.5% for boys). Girls were more likely than boys to have sent (11.5% for girls vs. 7.1% for boys) and received image-based sexts (36.2% for girls vs. 31.6%

TABLE 11.1 Descriptive data of all respondents who had at least engaged once in the respective types of sexting in the six months prior to the study. The two columns on the right display the prevalence rates of sexting according to the sex of the participants

Type of sexting behavior	n (%) total respondents who had experienced the behavior	n (%) male respondents who had experienced the behavior	n (%) female respondents who had experienced the behavior
Image-based sexting items			
Sent a sext	247 (9.6%)	79 (7.1%)	168 (11.5%)
Someone sent a sext of themselves to me	878 (34.2%)	351 (31.6%)	527 (36.2%)
Image-based sexual abuse items			
Someone persisted or pressured me to send a sext to that person	280 (10.9%)	39 (3.5%)	241 (16.6%)
I have forwarded a sext of someone else or showed it to other people, or posted it online	171 (6.7%)	94 (8.5%)	77 (5.3%)
Adult online sexual solicitation			
An adult asked me to send a sext	247 (9.6%)	43 (3.8%)	204 (13.9%)
An adult sent me a sext	400 (15.5%)	141 (12.6%)	259 (17.7%)

for boys) and experienced pressure to send an image-based sext (16.6% for girls vs. 3.5% for boys). Girls were also more likely than boys to have received a request to send (13.9% for girls vs. 3.8% for boys) and more likely to have received an unsolicited image-based sext from an adult (17.7% for girls vs. 12.6% for boys).

Discussion

With this chapter, we have contributed to a better understanding of image-based sexting and sexual abuse among early adolescents. The study's results show that image-based sexting, as a digital form of sexual communication, can start at a relatively early age, increases as adolescents grow

TABLE 11.2 Logistic regression models for different forms of sexting behaviors

Predictor	Sent a sexting picture		Received a sexting picture		Pressured to engage in sexting		Perpetration of non-consensual forwarding	
	B (S.E.)	Exp (B) [95% CI]	B (S.E.)	Exp (B) [95% CI]	B (S.E.)	Exp (B) [95% CI]	B (S.E.)	Exp (B) [95% CI]
Constant	-10.49 (1.12)	.00***	-10.03 (.72)	.00***	-11.86 (1.11)	.00***	-11.74 (1.35)	.00***
Sex (ref = male)	.53 (.14)	1.69 [1.28–2.25]***	.20 (.09)	1.22 [1.03–1.45]*	1.72 (.18)	5.59 [3.93–7.95]***	-.54 (.16)	.58[0.42–0.80]***
Age	.41 (.08)	1.51 [1.29–1.76]***	.48 (.05)	1.61 [1.46–1.78]***	.43 (.08)	1.54 [1.32–1.78]***	.47 (.09)	1.60 [1.34–1.92]***
Amount of internet use	.53 (.11)	1.70 [1.36–2.13]***	.64 (.07)	1.90 [1.66–2.18]***	.61 (.11)	1.84 [1.47–2.29]***	.66 (.14)	1.94 [1.47–2.57]***

*$p \leq .05$; ** $p \leq .01$; *** $p \leq .001$; CI = Confidence Interval.

TABLE 11.3 Logistic regression models for adult online sexual solicitation

Predictor	Being asked by an adult to send a sext		An adult sent a sext to the participant	
	B (S.E.)	Exp (B) [95% CI]	B (S.E.)	Exp (B) [95% CI]
Constant	-9.91 (1.13)	.00***	-7.16 (.89)	.00***
Sex (ref = male)	1.42 (.17)	4.16 [2.95–5.85]***	.41 (.11)	1.51 [1.20–1.89]***
Age	.26 (.08)	1.29 [1.11–1.51]***	.19 (.06)	1.20 [1.07–1.36]**
Amount of internet use	.72 (.12)	2.05 [1.62–2.60]***	.62 (.09)	1.85 [1.54–2.22]***

*p ≤ .05; **p ≤ .01; *** p ≤ .001; CI = Confidence Interval.

older, and that a considerable minority of early adolescents have experienced forms of image-based sexual abuse. These findings underscore the importance of sexual education focusing on the online behaviors and experiences of youth from an early age. Currently, there are almost no evidence-based educational resources available that teach adolescents about safer sexting practices. Safer sexting education should focus on teaching adolescents how to navigate the risks and to deal with pressure and requests for image-based sexts from peers, romantic partners, and adults. Such resources could be integrated in existing relational and sexual education programs (Madigan et al., 2018).

Moreover, such education programs should recognize the gendered experiences of image-based sexting and sexual abuse, and the sexual double standards in which such experiences are rooted. Our study found that boys are more likely to non-consensually forward an image-based sext, which aligns with prior research indicating how boys gain status in peer groups by asserting the possession and non-consensual distribution of girls' sexting messages (Ringrose et al., 2013). Girls, on the other hand, are expected to safeguard their own sexual reputation, while, at the same time, still needing to be sexually available to boys. Indeed, our findings show how girls were more likely to both send a sext and receive a sext, as well as experience pressure to engage in these sexting behaviors. These findings also align with prior research (Ringrose et al., 2022; Gámez-Guadix et al., 2018).

Several avenues for future research remain. First, our study was primarily descriptive to first gauge the prevalence of these behaviors. Future research should adopt a more theory-driven approach to gain a deeper understanding of the antecedents and consequences of engaging in image-based sexting and experiencing image-based sexual abuse during early adolescence. Using theoretical frameworks like the Differential Susceptibility to Media Effects Model (Valkenburg & Peter, 2013), future studies could explore factors that may place adolescents at risk of experiencing negative outcomes from these behaviors. The model allows for a detailed understanding of how dispositional, developmental, and social factors impact engagement in sexting. Furthermore, it would be a suitable framework to study how individuals' various response states can affect their responses to being a bystander of image-based sexual abuse.

Conclusion

This chapter explored the prevalence of image-based sexting experiences among early to middle adolescents, finding that approximately one in ten teens sent such sexts, and more than a third received them. Boys were more likely than girls to non-consensually forward an image-based sext, and girls were more likely to send or receive image-based sexts as well as experience image-based sexual abuse and adult sexual solicitation. Overall, these findings suggest that educational and prevention efforts focused on helping adolescents avoid image-based sexting may need to be specifically tailored to sex differences.

References

Bindesbøl Holm Johansen, K., Pedersen, B. M., & Tjørnhøj-Thomsen, T. (2019). Visual gossiping: non-consensual 'nude' sharing among young people in Denmark. *Culture, Health & Sexuality*, 21(9), 1029–1044. https://doi.org/10.1080/13691058.2018.1534140

Choi, H. J., Mori, C., Van Ouytsel, J., Madigan, S., & Temple, J. R. (2019). Adolescent sexting involvement over 4 years and associations with sexual activity. *Journal of Adolescent Health*, 65(6), 738–744. https://doi.org/10.1016/j.jadohealth.2019.04.026

Courtice, E. L., & Shaughnessy, K. (2021). Four problems in sexting research and their solutions. *Sexes*, 2(4), 415–432. https://doi.org/10.3390/sexes2040033

Gámez-Guadix, M., De Santisteban, P., & Alcazar, M. Á. (2018). The construction and psychometric properties of the questionnaire for online sexual solicitation and interaction of minors with adults. *Sexual Abuse*, 30(8), 975–991. https://doi.org/10.1177/1079063217724766

Huntington, C., & Rhoades, G. (2021). Associations of sexting with dating partners with adolescents' romantic relationship behaviors and attitudes. *Sexual and Relationship Therapy*, 38(4), 780–795. https://doi.org/10.1080/14681994.2021.1931096

Madigan, S., Ly, A., Rash, C. L., Van Ouytsel, J., & Temple, J. R. (2018). Prevalence of multiple forms of sexting behavior among youth: a systematic review and meta-analysis. *JAMA Pediatrics*, 172(4), 327–335. https://doi.org/10.1001/jamapediatrics.2017.5314

Maes, C., Van Ouytsel, J., & Vandenbosch, L. (2023). Victim blaming and non-consensual forwarding of sexts among late adolescents and young adults. *Archives of Sexual Behavior*, *52*(4), 1767–1783. https://doi.org/10.1007/s10508-023-02537-2

Maes, C., & Vandenbosch, L. (2022). Physically distant, virtually close: Adolescents' sexting behaviors during a strict lockdown period of the COVID-19 pandemic. *Computers in Human Behavior*, *126*, 107033. https://doi.org/10.1016/j.chb.2021.107033

Mitchell, K. J., Finkelhor, D., Jones, L. M., & Wolak, J. (2012). Prevalence and characteristics of youth sexting: A national study. *Pediatrics*, *129*(1), 13–20. https://doi.org/10.1542/peds.2011-1730

Paat, Y.-F., & Markham, C. (2021). Digital crime, trauma, and abuse: Internet safety and cyber risks for adolescents and emerging adults in the 21st century. *Social Work in Mental Health*, *19*(1), 18–40. https://doi.org/10.1080/15332985.2020.1845281

Patchin, J. W., & Hinduja, S. (2020). Sextortion among adolescents: Results from a national survey of U.S. youth. *Sexual Abuse*, *32*(1), 30–54. https://doi.org/10.1177/1079063218800469

Pampati, S., Lowry, R., Moreno, M. A., Rasberry, C. N., & Steiner, R. J. (2020). Having a sexual photo shared without permission and associated health risks: A snapshot of nonconsensual sexting. *JAMA Pediatrics*, *174*(6), 618–619. https://doi.org/10.1001/jamapediatrics.2020.0028

Pew Research Center. (2018, May). *Teens, Social Media and Technology 2018*. Retrieved from: https://www.pewresearch.org/internet/2018/05/31/teens-social-media-technology-2018/

Ringrose, J., Harvey, L., Gill, R., & Livingstone, S. (2013). Teen girls, sexual double standards and 'sexting': Gendered value in digital image exchange. *Feminist Theory*, *14*(3), 305–323. https://doi.org/10.1177/1464700113499853

Ringrose, J., Milne, B., Mishna, F., Regehr, K., & Slane, A. (2022). Young people's experiences of image-based sexual harassment and abuse in England and Canada: Toward a feminist framing of technologically facilitated sexual violence. *Women's Studies International Forum*, *93*, 102615. https://doi.org/10.1016/j.wsif.2022.102615

Valkenburg, P. M., & Peter, J. (2013). The differential susceptibility to media effects model. *Journal of Communication*, *63*(2), 221–243. https://doi.org/10.1111/jcom.12024

van de Bongardt, D., de Graaf, H., Reitz, E., & Deković, M. (2014). Parents as moderators of longitudinal associations between sexual peer norms and Dutch adolescents' sexual initiation and intention. *Journal of Adolescent Health*, *55*(3), 388–393. https://doi.org/10.1016/j.jadohealth.2014.02.017

Van Ouytsel, J., Van Gool, E., Ponnet, K., & Walrave, M. (2014). Brief report: The association between adolescents' characteristics and engagement in sexting. *Journal of Adolescence*, *37*(8), 1387–1391. https://doi.org/10.1016/j.adolescence.2014.10.004

Van Ouytsel, J., Walrave, M., De Marez, L., Vanhaelewyn, B., & Ponnet, K. (2021). Sexting, pressured sexting and image-based sexual abuse among a weighted-sample of heterosexual and LGB-youth. *Computers in Human Behavior*, *117*, 106630. https://doi.org/10.1016/j.chb.2020.106630

Van Ouytsel, J., Walrave, M., & Ponnet, K. (2019). Sexting within adolescents' romantic relationships: How is it related to perceptions of love and verbal conflict? *Computers in Human Behavior, 97*, 216–221. https://doi.org/10.1016/j.chb.2019.03.029

Vanden Abeele, M., Campbell, S. W., Eggermont, S., & Roe, K. (2014). Sexting, mobile porn use, and peer group dynamics: Boys' and girls' self-perceived popularity, need for popularity, and perceived peer pressure. *Media Psychology, 17*(1), 6–33. https://doi.org/10.1080/15213269.2013.801725

Walrave, M., Ponnet, K., Van Ouytsel, J., Van Gool, E., Heirman, W., & Verbeek, A. (2015). Whether or not to engage in sexting: Explaining adolescent sexting behaviour by applying the prototype willingness model. *Telematics and Informatics, 32*(4), 796–808. https://doi.org/10.1016/j.tele.2015.03.008

Casas, J.A., Ojeda, M., Elipe, P., & Del Rey, R. (2019). Exploring which factors contribute to teens' participation in sexting. *Computers in Human Behavior, 100*, 60-69. https://doi.org/10.1016/j.chb.2019.06.010

12

PEERS VERSUS PIXELS

Teen Sexting as Influenced by Peer Norms
and Pornography Use

*Rebecca Lin Densley, McCall Booth, and
Jane Shawcroft*

Over the past two decades, the use of smartphone and social media has
shifted teens' sexual media practices. Adolescents can easily access sexually
explicit media via online pornography (Giordano et al., 2022) and no longer exclusively consume sexual content produced by media companies;
they also create and share content featuring their own and peers' bodies in
sexual ways. Sexting—the digital exchange of sexual messages in the form
of images, videos, or text—is a prime example of teen sexual media "pro-
sumption" (Weimann et al., 2014), wherein teens simultaneously produce
and consume media content.

Although approximately 25% of adolescents sext (Giordano et al., 2022),
it is often viewed as risky. Beginning in the 2010s, the United States' popular
press has portrayed teen sexting as dangerous by emphasizing extreme, but
rare, sexting outcomes such as child sex crime charges, pedophile grooming,
sextortion, and teen suicide (e.g., Wolak et al., 2018). Many scholars argue
that this discourse is fueled by society's discomfort with adolescent sexuality
and does not provide teens, parents, and policymakers with helpful information about likely sexting outcomes (Crofts et al., 2015).

Teen sexting outcomes are varied and, depending on one's views about
adolescent sexuality, could be considered problematic or part of normal
sexual development. For example, some studies link sexting to risky sexual
behaviors and negative psychosocial health (Kurup et al., 2022), while others associate sexting with increased connection in committed relationships
and girls taking pride in their bodies and sexuality (García-Gómez, 2017).
Given the range of outcomes, it is important to understand situations in
which sexting occurs and social factors that influence sexting to make

DOI: 10.4324/9781032648880-15

meaningful recommendations to teens, parents, and policymakers regarding this increasingly common behavior.

Adolescents engage in sexting for many reasons, including boredom, desire for attention or sex, connection with romantic partners, and coercion (Ojeda et al., 2022). Social norms—or socially expected standards of behavior—around sexting come from multiple sources and influence if and why adolescents choose to sext. For example, listening to sexually explicit music is associated with increased sexting for boys (Keenan-Kroff et al., 2023). Similarly, pornography is associated with sexting for both boys and girls (Giordano et al., 2022)—arguably because sexually explicit media can demonstrate and normalize sexual behaviors (Laporte et al., 2020). Teens of a similar age and social context (i.e. "peers") are also prominent sources of sexual social norms (Endendijk et al., 2022). Research has linked peer sexting to teen sexting (Maheux et al., 2020), and most adolescents report that their peers generally approve of sexting, especially within a trusting, consensual relationship (Burén et al., 2022).

This chapter will expand on previous research by examining the association between peer social norms (herein referred to as "peer norms"), pornography use, and teen sexting. By analyzing the role of pornography alongside peer norms, we acknowledge multiple factors likely promote or discourage teen sexting. This research is also the first of its kind to assess the influence of multiple types of peer norms on teen sexting.

Social cognitive theory and the triadic reciprocal model of causation

Bandura's social cognitive theory (SCT) has become a foundational framework for explaining the importance of observational learning (1986); however, this theory goes beyond modeling and imitation. The theory's triadic reciprocal model claims that personal factors (e.g., one's biology and thoughts), environmental factors (e.g., peers and media), and behavioral factors (one's personal behaviors) influence one another and create a unique context wherein certain behaviors are more or less likely to occur. This chapter uses the triadic model as a framework, recognizing that adolescent sexting behaviors are likely influenced by both personal (i.e., age and gender) and environmental factors (i.e., peer norms and pornography). Figure 12.1 illustrates how key variables in the current study fit within the model.

Peer norms

Adolescents' peers might be a key source where desires to sext originate. Social norms theory proposes that when a person believes that their peers

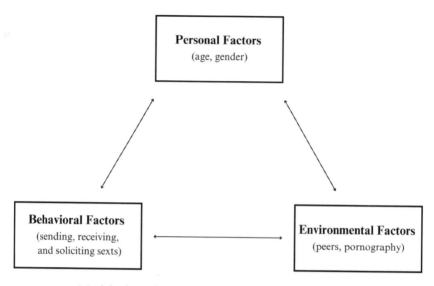

FIGURE 12.1   Model of triadic reciprocal causation in sexting context.

behave in a certain way, a "norm" is created and the behavior is often imitated (Cialdini et al., 1990). Importantly, social norms literature distinguishes two norm types—descriptive and injunctive. Descriptive norms refer to beliefs about the *prevalence* of behaviors among one's peers (e.g., how often one's friends sext) while injunctive norms refer to perceptions about one's peers' *approval* of behaviors (e.g., the belief that one's peers are okay with sexting). When adolescents believe that their peers are sexually active (descriptive norms) and approve of sexual activity (injunctive norms), they are more likely to be sexually active themselves. Similarly, adolescents' beliefs that peers disapprove of sex (injunctive norms) are associated with decreased sexual intercourse, fewer sexual partners, and intentions to remain abstinent (e.g., van de Bongardt et al., 2015).

Peers are an environmental factor within the SCT model of triadic reciprocal causation and might impact adolescents' sexting behavior through modeling (peers demonstrate sexting behaviors with or in the presence of each other), enactive experience (peers provide implicit messages by reacting to social situations where sexting occurs or is discussed), and direct tuition (peers share thoughts, experiences, and opinions about sexting with each other). Importantly, according to SCT, peers are salient models because people learn more from models they choose to associate with and can relate to (Bussey & Bandura, 1999). For this reason, closeness of peer relationships is important. Although distal peers (one's general peer group, but not close friends) may provide some cues for adolescents, close peers provide a more direct influence on developing teens (Paek & Gunther, 2007). Thus, intersecting both SCT and social norms theory, we predict:

H1: Descriptive sexting norms of close peers, but not distal peers, will be significantly associated with teens' sending (H1a), receiving (H1b), and soliciting sexts (H1c).

H2: Injunctive sexting norms of close peers, but not distal peers, will be significantly associated with teens' sending (H2a), receiving (H2b), and soliciting sexts (H2c).

Adolescent online pornography use

Online pornography is accessible, affordable, and anonymous (Cooper et al., 2000), which results in pornography use being common among adolescents. One recent study reported 68.4% of American adolescents have used pornography (Wright et al., 2020), with average age of first exposure being 12 years old (Robb & Mann, 2023). Adolescents may encounter a wide range of pornography types online, each yielding different effects. For example, violent pornography use is linked to sexual aggression and teen dating violence (Ferguson & Hartley, 2022), while general pornography use is associated with teens' self-objectification and body comparison, reduced condom use, and permissive sexual attitudes (Maheux et al., 2021; Wright et al., 2020). Furthermore, more than half of teens who use porn report having tried something in person they first saw in pornography (Rothman & Adhia, 2015).

Within SCT's model, media modeling is an influential environmental factor. Unfortunately, pornography frequently portrays risky sex practices, with little attention given to preventative measures for safe sex (Miller & McBain, 2022). Furthermore, in regions like North America, cultural taboos surrounding adolescent sexuality limit discussions of healthy sexual practices, which may result in pornography's sexual scripts remaining unchallenged (Ward et al., 2022). SCT suggests that when adolescents consume pornography, actors model sexual behaviors adolescents internalize and later exemplify in their own sexual practices, including sexting (Giordano et al., 2022). As such, we predict:

H3: Adolescent pornography use will be significantly associated with teens' sending (H3a), receiving (H3b), and soliciting sexts (H3c).

The role of gender

Although research demonstrates that sexting behaviors are linked to teen pornography use regardless of gender (Giordano et al., 2022), some studies have found that boys are more strongly influenced than girls by sexual media messages (Keenan-Kroff et al., 2023). Scholars attribute this gender moderation effect to the sexual double standard (Milhausen & Herold, 2002) prevalent in media and society, wherein male sexual behavior is rewarded while female sexual behavior is stigmatized. Boys consume more pornography than girls (Peter & Valkenburg, 2016), and common scripts presented in pornography focus on men's sexual pleasure, using women as instruments to achieve men's sexual satisfaction or to be collected and used for sexual purposes (Braithwaite et al., 2015). No research of which we are aware examines the moderating role of gender in the association between adolescent pornography use and sexting, we pose the question:

RQ1: Will adolescents' sending (RQ1a), receiving (RQ1b) and soliciting (RQ1c) sexts be moderated by gender such that boys who frequently use pornography will be more likely to sext than girls?

Magnitude of associations

Although we predict that peer norms and pornography use will be associated with sexting behaviors, the magnitude of these associations is unclear. Some research suggests that peers more strongly influence teens' sexual behaviors than media (Ferguson et al., 2017), while other studies emphasize the uniquely compelling nature of sexual media in its ability to shape sexual attitudes and behaviors (Laporte et al., 2020). As such, we pose the question:

RQ2: Will peer norms about sexting or pornography use be more strongly associated with teens' sending (RQ2a), receiving (RQ2b), and soliciting sexts (RQ2c)?

Method

Participants

The researchers' university Institutional Review Board granted approval prior to data collection, and the study was funded by university research funds. Participants for the online survey included 690 adolescents ages 15–18 (M = 16.12, SD = .93, 51.4% identified as female) recruited via Qualtrics' online participant pool across four main regions of the United States. Quota sampling yielded a sample reflecting U.S. census race and ethnicity rates: 63.9% White, 12.2% Black/African American, 12.9% Hispanic, 4.1% Asian, 2.2% Native American or Alaska Native, 1.3% Hawaiian or Pacific Islander, and 3.5% other race. Parents were given study information and provided consent for their teens to participate. Parents were then invited to give the adolescent privacy for the remainder of the survey. From there, adolescents were given study information and provided their assent before completing the survey.

Measures

Adolescents reported how often they used pornography, ranging from never (1) to several times a day (7), ($M = 2.93$, $SD = 1.37$). They also reported how often they sent, received, and solicited (i.e., asked someone to send) sexually explicit messages or pictures via cell phone within the past 12 months, ranging from never (1) to several times a day (7), (sent: $M = 1.51$, $SD = 1.03$; received: $M = 2.25$, $SD = 1.26$; solicited: $M = 1.43$, $SD = 1.02$) (see Table 12.1). All participants were asked how often their "guy friends" and "girl friends" sext (close descriptive norms: $M = 3.10$, $SD = 1.67$, $\alpha = .88$) and how often "a typical guy" and "a typical girl" of their age sext (distal descriptive norms: $M = 3.62$, $SD = 1.60$, $\alpha = .90$), ranging from never (1) to several times a day (7). In addition, they were asked whether "most of your friends," "your best friend," and "your boyfriend/girlfriend" would approve of them sexting (close injunctive norms: $M = 2.52$, $SD = 1.05$, $\alpha = .89$) and whether "most girls" and "most guys" of their age would approve of them sexting (distal injunctive norms: $M = 2.94$, $SD = .99$, $\alpha = .80$), ranging from strongly disapprove (1) to strongly approve (5). Finally, participants reported their gender, age, and race. For full measures, see Measurement Appendix.

TABLE 12.1 Adolescents' engagement in sexting behaviors in the last 12 months

	Overall		Males		Females	
	n	%	n	%	n	%
Sent a Sext	178	25.8	96	28.7	82	23.0
Received a Sext	356	51.6	183	54.6	173	48.7
Solicited a Sext	151	21.9	94	28.1	57	16.0

Note: This table shows participants who selected any response other than "never" for the sexting frequency questions.

Results

Hypotheses and research questions were tested with ordinal logistic regression analysis (Table 12.2), wherein three ordered models (one for each sexting behavior) were estimated to determine whether control variables, peer norm types, pornography use, and the interaction between gender and pornography use accounted for significant variance in frequency of sexting behaviors. Together, the predictors accounted for a significant amount of variance in the outcome likelihood ratio for sending sexts [$\chi^2(9) = 275.26$, $p < .001$], receiving sexts [$\chi^2(9) = 402.43$, $p < .001$], and soliciting sexts [$\chi^2(9) = 212.18$, $p < .001$].

Descriptive norms of close peers were significantly, independently associated with sending, receiving, and soliciting sexts, and descriptive norms of distal peers were not significantly associated with any sexting behaviors. Thus, H1 was confirmed. The injunctive norms of close peers were significantly, independently associated with sending, receiving, and soliciting sexts, and the injunctive norms of distal peers were significantly, independently associated with receiving sexts, partially confirming H2. In support

TABLE 12.2 Results of ordinal logistic regression analyses for sending, receiving, and soliciting sexts

	Sending a Sext		Receiving a Sext		Soliciting a Sext	
	B (SE)	OR	B (SE)	OR	B (SE)	OR
Predictors						
Gender (ref = female)	.46 (.40)	1.58	.38 (.32)	1.46	.46 (.44)	1.59
Age	.25 (.12)	1.29	.13 (.10)	1.14	.38 (.13)**	1.14
Race (ref = White)	-.41 (.21)*	.66	-.18 (.17)	.84	.01 (.21)	1.01
Close descriptive norms	.55 (.11)***	1.73	.63 (.09)***	1.88	.24 (.11)*	1.27
Distal descriptive norms	-.05 (.12)	.96	-.13 (.09)	.88	.15 (.12)	1.17
Close injunctive norms	.73 (.15)***	2.08	.28 (.12)*	1.32	.59 (.15)***	1.34
Distal injunctive norms	.09 (.18)	1.09	.42 (.13)**	1.16	-.02 (.19)	.68
Pornography use	.74 (.24)**	2.09	.91 (.23)***	1.60	.63 (.27)*	1.02
Gender × Porn use	-.19 (.14)	.63	-.20 (.13)	.64	-.03 (.16)	.72
McFadden's psuedo-R^2	.223		.221		.190	

*$p \le .05$. **$p \le .01$. ***$p \le .001$.

of H3, pornography use frequency was significantly, independently associated with sending, receiving, and soliciting sexts. The interaction between pornography use frequency and gender was not significant for any sexting behaviors (RQ1). Finally, the regression coefficients for pornography use were higher than peer norms for all three sexting behaviors (RQ2).

Discussion

This study explored adolescent sexting in the context of two key socializers: peers and pornography. We found that both descriptive norms (beliefs about prevalence of peers' sexting) and injunctive norms (beliefs about peers' approval of sexting) of close peers were significantly associated with teens' sending, receiving, and soliciting sexts. This highlights the important role an adolescent's close peer group, as opposed to one's peers in general, plays in their sexting behaviors, which is consistent with previous research in other contexts (van de Bongardt et al., 2015). As such, parents and educators who aim to engage in productive conversations about teen sexting would be wise to recognize that peer groups vary in their sexting attitudes and behaviors and close friends are likely more influential than stories about sexting a teen may overhear at school or in the news. Such stakeholders will be better able to tailor their messages to teens if they ask what kinds of information and experiences about sexting have been shared between friends. Of note, the only significant association for distal peers was between injunctive norms and receiving sexts, which suggests that adolescents may deal with unsolicited sexts from distal peers who feel positively about sexting. Indeed, studies have shown that many adolescents receive unwanted sexts (Barroso et al., 2023). This finding points to the importance of discussing sexual consent with teens as well as teaching them what they can and should do when they receive unwanted sexts.

Second, we found that adolescent pornography use was associated with sending, receiving, and soliciting sexts and that the magnitude of these associations was larger than for peer norms. Peers are a key influence on adolescent beliefs and behaviors (van de Bongardt et al., 2015), so it may come as a surprise that pornography use presented a stronger relationship to sexting. Mass media has been called a sexual "super peer" (Brown et al., 2005) and, as conversations in the United States around adolescent sexuality are still met with social taboo (Ward et al., 2022), teens may consider pornography more reliable and accessible for sexual information than their peers (Seifadin & Wakeshi, 2019). Importantly, this study also demonstrated that the link between pornography use and sexting is not significantly stronger for boys than girls. In the present study, more boys (58%) than girls (26%) reported pornography use, but ultimately pornography relates to sexting behaviors for boys and girls alike. One limitation of our data is that it is limited to those who identify as either male or female, as none of our participants identified as non-binary; however, findings suggest that adolescents who regularly consume pornography may use sexting to imitate behaviors from pornography. After all, pornography, like sexting, captures sexual activity in a digital format and is most often viewed/ shared on phones (Pornhub, 2023).

Although similar in many ways, there are differentiating factors that adolescents, caregivers, educators, and policymakers should consider regarding pornography use and sexting, as certain behaviors can result in legal ramifications for teens in the United States. For example, one key issue with adolescent sexting is consent. Sexts shared between adolescents are not always consensual (Barroso et al., 2023), and sexts distributed without permission are considered "revenge porn," potentially resulting in misdemeanor or felony charges for minors in most U.S. states (Jeter, 2021). As pornography may not clearly demonstrate sexual consent, the connection between porn and sexting could be especially problematic for teens who do not think critically about messages in pornography. Furthermore, one important difference between most pornography and adolescent sexts is the age of subjects in the explicit material. Unlike most mainstream pornography, sexts created and shared among adolescents portray minors engaging in sexual acts and therefore are often considered child pornography (Strasburger et al., 2019). Unfortunately, important conversations distinguishing pornography from sexting—and encouraging adolescents to consider consent and age when sexting—may not be occurring. In fact, teens report turning to pornography for information about sex due to limited access to reliable and credible sexual information elsewhere (Seifadin & Wakeshi, 2019). Like all media content, however, pornography is merely a media construction, not a reflection of reality. As such, it is important to encourage adolescents to think critically about the sexual scripts they encounter in pornography, a concept called "porn literacy" (Rothman et al., 2018). Porn-literate adolescents would scrutinize whether pornography messages promote healthy sexual development and consider ways in which pornography and sexting differ, especially among minors. Furthermore, parents and educators should explicitly teach principles of healthy sexual relationships (e.g., boundaries, consent, or disease prevention) to counteract problematic sexual information provided by peers and pornography and help adolescents recognize that certain behaviors seen in pornography could result in negative outcomes if imitated in sexting.

Ultimately, adolescence is a time of discovery and emerging sexuality. It is important to empower adolescents by providing them with clear and useful sexual information and encouraging them to think critically about all media content—pornography included. Future research ought to explore patterns of adolescent sexting and examine whether and how teens differentiate pornography from sexting. As suggested in our study, there is a need for clear consent and boundaries in digital sexual relationships. Parents and educators can promote adolescents' healthy sexual development by ensuring that discussions of pornography and sexting highlight the importance of consent and sexual health.

References

Bandura, A. (1986). *Social Foundations of thought and action: A social cognitive theory.* Englewood Cliffs, NJ: Prentice-Hall.

Barroso, R., Marinho, A. R., Figueiredo, P., Ramião, E., Silva, A. S. (2023). Consensual and non-consensual sexting behaviors in adolescence: A systematic review. *Adolescent Research Review, 8,* 1–20. https://doi.org/10.1007/s40894-022-00199-0

Braithwaite, S. R., Coulson, G., Keddington, K., & Fincham, F. D. (2015). The influence of pornography on sexual scripts and hooking up among emerging adults in college. *Archives of Sexual Behavior, 44*(1), 111–123. https://doi.org/10.1007/s10508-014-0351-x

Brown, J. D., Halpern, C. T., & L'Engle, K. L. (2005). Mass media as a sexual super peer for early maturing girls. *Journal of Adolescent Health, 36*(5), 420–427. https://doi.org/10.1016/j.jadohealth.2004.06.003

Burén, J., Holmqvist Gattario, K., & Lunde, C. (2022). What do peers think about sexting? Adolescents' views of the norms guiding sexting behavior. *Journal of Adolescent Research, 37*(2), 221–249. https://doi.org/10.1177/07435584211014837

Bussey, K., & Bandura, A. (1999). Social cognitive theory of gender development and differentiation. *Psychological Review, 106*(4), 676.

Cialdini, R. B., Reno, R. R., & Kallgren, C. A. (1990). A focus theory of normative conduct: Recycling the concept of norms to reduce littering in public places. *Journal of Personality and Social Psychology, 58*(6), 1015. https://doi.org/10.1037/0022-3514.58.6.1015

Cooper, A., Delmonico, D. L., & Burg, R. (2000). Cybersex users, abusers, and compulsives: New findings and implications. *Sexual Addiction & Compulsivity: The Journal of Treatment and Prevention, 7*(1–2), 5–29. https://doi.org/10.1080/10720160008400205

Crofts, T., Lee, M., McGovern, A., & Milivojevic, S. (2015). Making sense of sexting. In T. Crofts, M. Lee, A. McGovern, & S. Milivojevic (eds.), *Sexting and young people* (pp. 161–178). Palgrave Macmillan UK. https://doi.org/10.1057/9781137392817_11

Endendijk, J. J., Deković, M., Vossen, H., van Baar, A. L., & Reitz, E. (2022). Sexual double standards: Contributions of sexual socialization by parents, peers, and the media. *Archives of Sexual Behavior, 51*(3), 1721–1740. https://doi.org/10.1007/s10508-021-02088-4

Ferguson, C. J., & Hartley, R. D. (2022). Pornography and sexual aggression: Can meta-analysis find a link? *Trauma, Violence & Abuse, 23*(1), 278–287. https://doi.org/10.1177/1524838020942754

Ferguson, C. J., Nielsen, R. K., & Markey, P. M. (2017). Does sexy media promote teen sex? A meta-analytic and methodological review. *Psychiatric Quarterly, 88*, 349–358. https://doi.org/10.1007/s11126-016-9442-2

García-Gómez, A. (2017). Teen girls and sexual agency: Exploring the intrapersonal and intergroup dimensions of sexting. *Media, Culture & Society, 39*(3), 391–407. https://doi.org/10.1177/0163443716683789

Giordano, A. L., Schmit, M. K., Clement, K., Potts, E. E., & Graham, A. R. (2022). Pornography use and sexting trends among American adolescents: Data to inform school counseling programming and practice. *Professional School Counseling, 26*(1). https://doi.org/10.1177/2156759X221137287

Jeter, L. (2021, November 16). *An update on the legal landscape of revenge porn.* National Association of Attorneys General. https://www.naag.org/attorney-general-journal/an-update-on-the-legal-landscape-of-revenge-porn/

Keenan-Kroff, S. L., Coyne, S. M., Shawcroft, J., Sheppard, J. A., James, S. L., Ehrenreich, S. E., & Underwood, M. (2023). Associations between sexual music lyrics and sexting across adolescence. *Computers in Human Behavior, 140*, 107562. https://doi.org/10.1016/j.chb.2022.107562

Kurup, A. R., George, M. J., Burnell, K., & Underwood, M. K. (2022). A longitudinal investigation of observed adolescent text-based sexting and adjustment. *Research on Child and Adolescent Psychopathology, 50*(4), 431–445. https://doi.org/10.1007/s10802-021-00850-9

Laporte, H., Rousseau, A., & Eggermont, S. (2020). Effects of media on sexual behaviors. In *The international encyclopedia of media psychology* (pp. 1–12). John Wiley & Sons, Ltd. https://doi.org/10.1002/9781119011071.iemp0110

Maheux, A. J., Evans, R., Widman, L., Nesi, J., Prinstein, M. J., & Choukas-Bradley, S. (2020). Popular peer norms and adolescent sexting behavior. *Journal of Adolescence, 78*, 62–66. https://doi.org/10.1016/j.adolescence.2019.12.002

Maheux, A. J., Roberts, S. R., Evans, R., Widman, L., & Choukas-Bradley, S. (2021). Associations between adolescents' pornography consumption and self-objectification, body comparison, and body shame. *Body Image 37*, 89–93. https://doi.org/10.1016/j.bodyim.2021.01.014

Milhausen, R. R., & Herold, E. S. (2002). Reconceptualizing the sexual double standard. *Journal of Psychology & Human Sexuality, 13*(2), 63–83. https://doi.org/10.1300/J056v13n02_05

Miller, D. J., & McBain, K. A. (2022). The content of contemporary, mainstream pornography: A literature review of content analytic studies. *American Journal of Sexuality Education, 17*(2), 219–256. https://doi.org/10.1080/15546128.2021.2019648

Ojeda, M., Dodaj, A., Sesar, K., & Del Rey, R. (2022). "Some voluntarily and some under pressure": Conceptualization, reasons, attitudes, and consequences of sexting among adolescents. *Telematics and Informatics, 75*, 101891. https://doi.org/10.1016/j.tele.2022.101891

Paek, H. J., & Gunther, A. C. (2007). How peer proximity moderates indirect media influence on adolescent smoking. *Communication Research, 34*(4), 407–432. https://doi.org/10.1177/0093650207302785

Peter, J., & Valkenburg, P. M. (2016). Adolescents and pornography: A review of 20 years of research. *The Journal of Sex Research*, *53*(4–5), 509–531. https://doi.org/10.1080/00224499.2016.1143441

Pornhub. (2023, December 9). *Year in review—Pornhub insights*. https://www.pornhub.com/insights/2023-year-in-review

Robb, M. B., & Mann, S. (2023). *2022 Teens and Pornography*. Common Sense Media.

Rothman, E. F., & Adhia, A. (2015). Adolescent pornography use and dating violence among a sample of primarily Black and Hispanic, urban-residing, underage youth. *Behavioral Sciences (Basel, Switzerland)*, *6*(1), 1. https://doi.org/10.3390/bs6010001

Rothman, E. F., Adhia, A., Christensen, T. T., Paruk, J., Alder, J., & Daley, N. (2018). A pornography literacy class for youth: Results of a feasibility and efficacy pilot study. *American Journal of Sexuality Education*, *13*(1), 1–17. https://doi.org/10.1080/15546128.2018.1437100

Seifadin, A. S., & Wakeshi, W. M. (2019). Exposure to sexually explicit materials and its association with sexual behaviors of Ambo University undergraduate students, 2018. *Ethiopian Journal of Health Sciences*, *29*(4), 461–470. https://doi.org/10.4314/ejhs.v29i4.7

Strasburger, V. C., Zimmerman, H., Temple, J. R., & Madigan, S. (2019). Teenagers, Sexting, and the Law. *Pediatrics*, *143*(5), e20183183. https://doi.org/10.1542/peds.2018-3183

van de Bongardt, D., Reitz, E., Sandfort, T., & Deković, M. (2015). A meta-analysis of the relations between three types of peer norms and adolescent sexual behavior. *Personality and Social Psychology Review*, *19*(3), 203–234. https://doi.org//10.1177/1088868314544223

Ward, L. M., Rosenscruggs, D., & Aguinaldo, E. R. (2022). A scripted sexuality: Media, gendered sexual scripts, and their impact on our lives. *Current Directions in Psychological Science*, *31*(4), 369–374. https://doi.org/10.1177/09637214221101072

Weimann, G., Weiss-Blatt, N., Mengistu, G., Tregerman, M. M., & Oren, R. (2014). Reevaluating "The End of Mass Communication?" *Mass Communication & Society*, *17*(6), 803–829. https://doi.org/10.1080/15205436.2013.851700

Wolak, J., Finkelhor, D., Walsh, W., & Treitman, L. (2018). Sextortion of minors: characteristics and dynamics. *The Journal of Adolescent Health*, *62*(1), 72–79. https://doi.org/10.1016/j.jadohealth.2017.08.014

Wright, P. J., Herbenick, D., & Paul, B. (2020). Adolescent condom use, parent-adolescent sexual health communication, and pornography: Findings from a U.S. probability sample. *Health Communication*, *35*(13), 1576–1582. https://doi.org/10.1080/10410236.2019.1652392

13

TECHNOLOGY-FACILITATED SEXUAL VIOLENCE AMONG ADOLESCENTS

Prevalence, Age and Gender Differences, Changes Over Time, and Mental Health Outcomes

Jone Martínez-Bacaicoa, Mariana Alonso-Fernández, and Manuel Gámez-Guadix

In 2016 in Spain, five men took a young woman to the entrance of a building and sexually assaulted her. During the trial, video footage recorded by the attackers, showing the apparently passive victim, was presented as evidence by the defense, alleging that the woman had consented to the sexual assaults. This case, known as *La Manada*, or the "wolf pack" case, sparked significant controversy in Spain and drew media attention to the culture of rape and the need for legal reforms (Aurrekoetxea-Casaus, 2020). Protests and demonstrations under the slogan *Yo sí te creo* (I believe you) spread throughout Spain, both in the online and offline realms, manifesting support for the victim and calling for justice (Idoiaga et al., 2020). Simultaneously, on the international stage, the emergence of the #MeToo movement in late 2017 empowered thousands of women to share their experiences with sexual misconduct facilitating widespread discussion of all forms of harassment and abuse faced by women (Hillstrom, 2018). However, it is important to note that during these events, the internet was also inundated with messages that promoted rape myths, which are false beliefs used to justify and excuse sexual violence, blame the victim, and minimize the seriousness of what had happened (Aurrekoetxea-Casaus, 2020).

This demonstrates how the social and digital realms are intertwined (Henry & Powell, 2015), especially for adolescents who have found in social media their fundamental tool for connection (Estébanez, 2018). This implies that, although information and communication technologies can serve as powerful tools for connecting with like-minded groups and establishing online support networks (Craig et al., 2023), they also give rise to

DOI: 10.4324/9781032648880-16

new systems of production and maintenance of hierarchies, behaviors, established roles in society, and traditional forms of violence (Donoso et al., 2017). In this context, there is a global growth in technology-facilitated sexual violence (TFSV), which refers to the use of digital technologies to perpetrate various harmful behaviors based on gender and sexuality (Henry & Powell, 2015). This umbrella term encompasses different behaviors, such as degrading comments or allusions related to someone's gender (i.e., gender-based violence) or sexual orientation (i.e., sexual orientation-based violence), aggressions motivated by the manifestation of behaviors discordant with assigned gender roles (i.e., gender role-based violence), the sending of nude images or unsolicited sexual messages (i.e., digital sexual harassment), threats or blackmail to share sexual images of an individual without their consent (e.g., sextortion), or the unauthorized distribution or publication of sexually explicit images of another person (i.e., nonconsensual sexting) (Gámez-Guadix, Sorrel et al., 2022; Powell & Henry, 2019).

Although these forms of violence may be interconnected (Gámez-Guadix, Sorrel et al., 2022), most studies have focused on analyzing them separately. This approach has made it challenging to gather comprehensive data on their overall incidence, limiting our understanding of the full scope of TFSV. However, existing evidence indicates that we are dealing with a widespread problem. Regarding sextortion, victimization rates range from 3.30% (Morelli et al., 2016) to 5% (Patchin & Hinduja, 2020), and even as high as 23% (Englander & McCoy, 2017). In the case of nonconsensual sexting, rates vary between 6% (Reed et al., 2019) and 24% (Englander & McCoy, 2017) among adolescents and young adults. These figures are even higher for other forms of TFSV, such as digital sexual harassment, for which victimization rates range from 10.9% (Donoso et al., 2017) to 15.4% (Hsieh et al., 2023), and 23% (Sklenarova et al., 2018), with rates peaking at 53% among female-only samples (Reed et al., 2019). Among adolescents identifying as sexual minorities, the rates also rise, with 45.2% experiencing digital sexual harassment, 41.1% facing online sexual orientation discrimination, and 28.4% reporting gender-based victimization (Gámez-Guadix & Íncera, 2021). Some evidence suggests that these rates may increase over the adolescent years as internet usage, exploration of sexuality, and adolescents' exposure to online risks increase (Gámez-Guadix, Sorrel et al., 2022). Rates may also vary by gender, with boys often identified as perpetrators and girls as victims, despite the potential for both genders to experience victimization (e.g., Powell & Henry, 2019). The prevalence of these forms of violence is worrisome because, while their visibility facilitates recognition among young people, it may lead to their normalization, perpetuating their occurrence (Martínez-Bacaicoa et al., 2024).

TFSV is a serious problem, with significant emotional, psychological, and sometimes physical consequences for the victims. These consequences range from a decrease in self-esteem and trust in others to symptoms of anxiety and depression and self-injurious behaviors and suicidal thoughts (Champion et al., 2022; Powell et al., 2018). Empirical evidence indicates that these consequences tend to be more harmful to those whom traditional gender roles place in a subordinate position (i.e., women and sexual minorities) (e.g., DeKeseredy et al., 2019) and for younger adolescents, who are in the process of social, psychological, and sexual development (Gámez-Guadix et al., 2018). However, despite the importance of analyzing and understanding the persistence of victimization in TFSV over time and its impact on adolescents, few studies have addressed this issue. Additionally, there is limited empirical evidence on whether the relationship between victimization and poorer mental health may vary depending on the gender and age of adolescents.

Present study

The present empirical study aims to fill the gaps in the literature and pursue the following objectives: (a) analyze the prevalence of the main types of TFSV among adolescents; (b) examine the differences in the prevalence of TFSV related to gender and age; (c) investigate the changes in TFSV victimization over one year; and (d) explore whether being a victim of TFSV is related to the presence of psychological symptoms (anxiety and depression) after one year, examining whether this relationship varies by victim gender and age. By addressing these objectives, we aim to contribute to a better understanding of TFSV and its implications for adolescent well-being.

Method

We conducted a longitudinal in-person survey among teens recruited from ten schools in Spain.

Participants

The initial sample was composed of 1,759 adolescents aged 12–16 years ($M = 13.85$; $SD = 1.2$). Among them, 902 (51.3%) were girls, 851 (48.4%) were boys, five (0.3%) were non-binary, and one (0.1%) did not indicate the gender. Most of the adolescents (89.7%) were heterosexual, 5.7% were bisexual, 1.7% were homosexual, 2% indicated having another sexual orientation, and 0.9% did not answer this question. Regarding birth countries, most participants were Spanish (87.83%), with smaller percentages from other Latin American (8.35%), European (1.14%), Asian (1.14%), African (0.7%), unspecified countries (0.74%), or North American (0.1%).

Procedure

Ten schools, selected randomly from a central region of Spain, participated in the study. The first data collection occurred between November 2019 and March 2020. Prior to commencement, letters were sent to parents requesting explicit approval for their children's participation, and adolescents received documentation affirming the voluntary nature of their involvement and ensuring confidentiality. Participants were informed of their right to skip questions or withdraw from the study without consequence. Questionnaires were completed individually in classrooms, with participants encouraged to seek clarification if needed. Following completion, participants were provided with written information on community counseling resources. The questionnaire required approximately 30-40 minutes for completion on both occasions. A unique code was assigned to each participant during the initial data collection to confidentially pair data collected one year later. Of the 1,767 adolescents initially enrolled, 897 completed measures again one year later. The study adhered to ethical standards outlined in the Declaration of Helsinki and received approval from the Ethics Committee of the Autonomous University of Madrid.

Funding for this study was provided by the Ministerio de Ciencia e Innovación (Spanish Government) grant PID2022-140195NB-I00 and the predoctoral contracts PRE2019-089729 and FPU21/01549.

Measures

Technology-facilitated sexual violence (TFSV) scales

Given the absence of instruments to assess TFSV, we developed a series of scales based on previous approaches to the constructs (e.g., Powell & Henry, 2019) and measures with good psychometric properties (Gámez-Guadix & Íncera, 2021). The content of the scales is provided in the Measurement Appendix. The internal consistency of the scales (Cronbach's alpha) was as follows: .84 at T1 and .83 at T2 for the gender-based violence scale, .87 at T1 and .88 at T2 for the gender role-based scale, .81 at T1 and .86 at T2 for the sexual orientation-based scale, .84 at T1 and .89 at T2 for the digital sexual harassment scale, .77 at T1 and .74 at T2 for the nonconsensual sexting scale, and .89 at T1 and .96 at T2 for the sextortion scale.

Mental health measures

Brief Symptom Inventory (BSI; Derogatis & Fitzpatrick, 2004). The depression and anxiety subscales of the BSI were used to evaluate mental health outcomes. In this sample, the internal consistency of the anxiety subscale was .87 at T1 and .90 at T2. The internal consistency of the depression subscale was .89 at T1 and .90 at T2. For more details about all measures described here, please see the Measurement Appendix.

Data analysis

To examine the prevalence of the victimization of different forms of TFSV, variables were dichotomized into "never" (0) and "one or more times" (1). Pearson's χ^2 test was used to assess gender and age differences, with age groups defined based on the legal age in Spain for accessing social networks (14 years). Spearman correlations were used to study the changes over time in TFSV victimization. Finally, the relationship between TFSV victimization and psychological outcomes one year later was explored using two linear regressions, with types of victimization as predictors and T2 anxiety and T2 depression as dependent variables. Gender, age, and psychological symptomatology at baseline were included as control variables. The proportion of missing values was below 5%; therefore, the listwise deletion method was employed to handle the missing data (Drechsler, 2015). Statistical analyses were conducted using SPSS software (Version 28).

Results

Prevalence of TFSV and gender and age differences

Table 13.1 presents the frequency of T1 victimization of the different types of TFSV in the past 12 months, along with age and gender differences. Approximately one-third (34.5%, $n = 604$) of the sample had experienced TFSV during the previous year. Digital sexual harassment emerged as the most prevalent form of TFSV (23.3%, $n = 408$), and sextortion was the least prevalent one (2.3%, $n = 40$). Gender analysis revealed significantly higher victimization among girls than boys (46.3% vs. 21.9%) except for sextortion.

Regarding age differences, the group aged 14–16 consistently experienced significantly higher rates of violence compared to the group aged

TABLE 13.1 Gender and age differences and the T1 prevalence of TFSV victimization

	Total	Gender			Age		
	N = 1,753	Girls n = 902	Boys n = 851	x^2	12–13 n = 988	14–16 n = 765	x^2
Gender-based violence	17.4%	26%	8.2%	91.908***	12.7%	23.5%	33.128***
Gender role-based violence	10.9%	16.1%	5.5%	47.806***	9.4%	12.9%	5.315*
Sexual orientation-based violence	6.1%	8.1%	3.9%	13.739***	3.7%	9%	21.064***
Digital sexual harassment	23.3%	33.8%	12.2%	113.469***	15.4%	33.6%	79.304***
Sextortion	2.3%	2.9%	1.6%	3.018	1.6%	3.1%	4.477*
Nonconsensual sexting	3.4%	4.6%	2.1%	7.899*	2.2%	4.8%	8.996**
Total	34.5%	46.3%	21.9%	116.240***	26.3%	45%	66.416***

Note: Prevalence refers to participants who reported having suffered some form of TFSV at least once in the last 12 months. $*p < .05$, $**p < .01$, $***p < .001$.

12–13 (45% vs. 26.3%). These age differences were consistent across all types of TFSV. Although older adolescents experienced more TFSV, the results also show that one in four 12- and 13-year-old adolescents have already experienced some type of victimization.

Changes over time in TFSV victimization

We analyzed the changes in various forms of TFSV victimization over a one-year follow-up period. The Spearman correlations between measures taken at baseline and one year later were .33 ($p < 0.01$) for gender-based victimization, .35 ($p < 0.01$) for gender role-based violence victimization, .42 ($p < 0.01$) for sexual orientation-based violence victimization, .44 ($p < 0.01$) for digital sexual harassment, .33 ($p < 0.01$) for sextortion victimization, and .33 ($p < 0.01$) for nonconsensual sexting victimization. These correlations showed a medium to large effect size and suggest some stability in TFSV experiences over time.

The relationship between TFSV victimization and mental health

Spearman correlations indicated a positive association between experiencing TFSV victimization and having more symptoms of anxiety and depression, both at baseline and one year later. Correlations ranged from .046 (*ns*) for nonconsensual sexting at T1 and the presence of anxious symptomatology at T2 to .397 ($p < .01$) for digital sexual harassment victimization at T1 and the presence of depressive symptomatology during that time.

To explore whether various forms of TFSV victimization at T1 predicted future anxiety and depression symptoms at T2, we conducted two hierarchical regression analyses (Table 13.2). In the initial step, we controlled for age, gender, and baseline psychological symptoms (utilizing T1 anxiety for cases where T2 anxiety was the criterion variable, and T1 depression for cases where T2 depression was the criterion variable). In the second step, we introduced the different forms of TFSV victimization at baseline to evaluate their predictive capacity for psychological symptomatology one year later. The result of these regression analyses indicates that T1 gender role-based violence ($\beta = .14$, $p < .001$) and T1 digital sexual harassment ($\beta = .10$, $p < .01$) predicted anxiety symptoms at T2. In addition, interactions were calculated to test the effects of gender and age. The PROCESS macro for SPSS was used to calculate and plot the interactions one by one. The interactions between gender and being a victim of gender-based violence were significant in predicting T2 anxiety ($\beta = -.25$, $p < .05$) and T2 depression ($\beta = -.25$, $p < .05$). The interaction between age and

TABLE 13.2 Linear regression models for the relationship between T1 technology-facilitated sexual victimization and T2 anxiety and T2 depression

	T2 Anxiety				T2 Depression			
	Step 1		Step 2		Step 1		Step 2	
	β	SE	β	SE	β	SE	β	SE
Age	-.01	.02	-.03	.03	.06	.03	.05	.03
Gender	-.27***	.06	-.23***	.06	-.22***	.06	-.19***	.06
T1 Anxiety/ depression	.44***	.03	.38***	.04	.48***	.03	.45***	.04
T1 Gender-based violence			-.03	.02			-.01	.03
T1 Gender role-based violence			.14***	.02			.05	.03
T1 Sexual orientation-based violence			.03	.05			.01	.05
T1 Digital sexual harassment			.10**	.03			.07	.03
T1 Sextortion			-.04	.13			.02	.14
T1 Nonconsensual sexting			-.02	.09			-.04	.09
R^2	.29		.31		.32		.34	

Note: 1 = girl, 2 = boy, $*p < .05$, $**p < .01$, $***p < .001$.

digital sexual harassment was significant in predicting anxiety ($\beta = -.10$, $p < .05$). The graphical representations of these interactions are shown in Figures 13.1–13.3. Figures 13.1 and 13.2 show that girls who experienced gender-based violence presented worse psychological symptoms (T2 anxiety and T2 depression) than boys. Regarding age, Figure 13.3 shows that the relationship between digital sexual harassment victimization and T2 anxiety was stronger for younger respondents.

Discussion

TFSV is a prevalent phenomenon that primarily affects girls. Approximately one in three adolescents experienced some form of TFSV in the past year. Compared to boys (around 22%), more than twice as many girls (roughly 46%) had been victims of some form of TFSV during the last year. The gendered nature of this issue is also evident in the impact TFSV has on victims. In our study, experiences of gender-based violence were

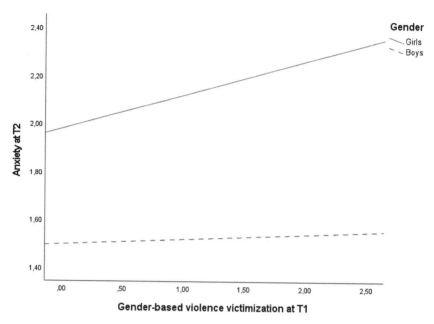

FIGURE 13.1 Moderating role of gender in the relationship between gender-based victimization and anxiety symptoms one year later.

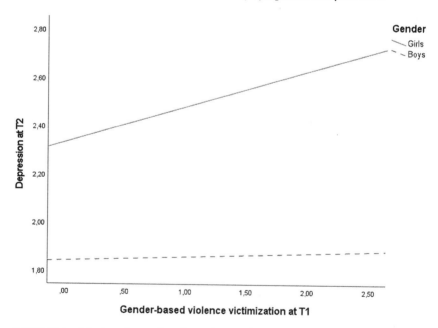

FIGURE 13.2 Moderating role of gender in the relationship between gender-based victimization and depression symptoms one year later.

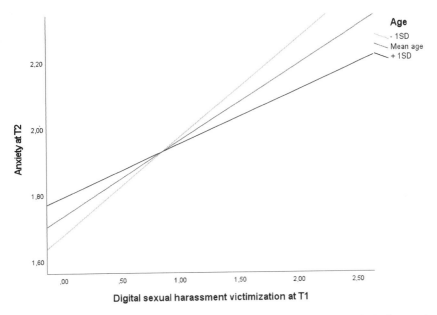

FIGURE 13.3   Moderating role of age in the relationship between digital sexual harassment victimization and anxiety symptoms one year later.

Note: SD = Standard Deviation.

linked to the presence of anxious and depressive symptoms one year after the TFSV aggression, especially in the case of girls. To understand these results, it is necessary to consider that online aggression can be permanent (hurtful comments can remain online indefinitely) and have a wide audience (many people can observe them), which can prolong the victims' suffering (Henry & Powell, 2015). Moreover, when the content of the aggression is misogynistic, as in gender-based violence, gender stereotypes may come into play, resulting in women being judged more harshly than men. This, in turn, may lead adolescent girls to avoid certain online spaces to prevent violence, ultimately widening the digital gender gap (Nadim & Fladmoe, 2021).

The findings of this study also indicate that age significantly influences the experience of TFSV victimization during adolescence. We consistently found that adolescents older than 14 had significantly higher rates of TFSV victimization. However, younger participants (12–13 years old) demonstrated greater long-term anxiety associated with experiencing digital sexual harassment. This may be related to the cognitive and emotional development of adolescents at different stages of puberty. As young people move through early to mid-adolescence, they experience significant physiological and emotional changes (Blakemore, 2012), potentially leading to further exploration of sexuality and increased exposure to online risks (Gámez-Guadix et al., 2016). Additionally, older adolescents, with more experience in online platforms, may be more exposed to different forms of TFSV. Nevertheless, their greater experience could also equip them with better strategies to navigate virtual violence and its consequences (Carcelén-García et al., 2023). In contrast, younger adolescents, less exposed to the online context, may find themselves more vulnerable to online violence, leading to increased psychological distress over time.

Moreover, our findings reveal significant correlations between the measurements of different forms of TFSV over one year, suggesting the potential recurrence of TFSV experiences. This underscores the need for early implementation of preventive interventions to equip adolescents with strategies to recognize and address risky situations and instances of TFSV as they begin using the Internet. Likewise, these interventions should address the gendered nature of TFSV and provide adolescents with a gender perspective to critically assess the misogyny that is being spread online. This is important because the internet is a socializing agent (Del Prete & Redon Pantoja, 2020), and many young people, whose identities are still developing, may end up normalizing behaviors that promote gender inequality.

Cultural variables that could affect TFSV

Social and cultural variables may have affected the results of the present study. Spain's culture has historically been characterized by traditional gender roles, such as the so-called "machismo" (Pérez-Martínez et al., 2021). However, Spanish society has experienced considerable progress in gender equality in the last two decades, catching up with other European countries. An illustrative instance is the aforementioned *La Manada* (wolf pack) case, which inundated the streets and the internet with expressions of outrage regarding the verdict and messages of support for the victim (Idoiaga et al., 2020). In this scenario, social media played a pivotal role in bringing the issue of consent in relationships to the forefront, exemplified by the hashtag *#NoesNo* (#NomeansNo), and advocating for both social and legislative changes (Aurrekoetxea-Casaus, 2020). The pressure exerted by the feminist movement was so profound that the Spanish Supreme Court eventually corrected the verdict and acknowledged that it was not a case of abuse but a case of rape (Rincón, 2019). This, in turn, led to significantly harsher sentences for all accused individuals and marked a shift in the Spanish social context. This case mirrors a social evolution that may have affected the rates of various forms of TFSV, which might be lower in Spain than in other cultural contexts.

Conclusion

In summary, this study provides compelling evidence for the prevalence of TFSV among adolescents and its association with mental health problems. Important gender and age differences in the prevalence of TFSV were identified, which highlights the need for gender- and age-specific preventive strategies. The findings suggest that TFSV tends to persist over time, which implies the need for early intervention to avoid chronicity. Prevention should consider cultural and social factors (e.g., gender norms), which may influence the prevalence and forms of TFSV. In addition, it is necessary to develop and implement prevention and support programs that address both TFSV and associated mental health problems and that promote respect and equality in online interactions. In conclusion, TFSV is a relevant problem that requires a holistic approach involving society, educators, parents, and adolescents to find a solution.

References

Aurrekoetxea-Casaus, M. (2020). San fermines# la manada case: An exploratory analysis of social support for victims of sexual violence on Twitter. *Computers in Human Behavior, 108,* 106299. https://doi.org/10.1016/j.chb.2020.106299

Blakemore, S.-J. (2012). Development of the social brain in adolescence. *Journal of the Royal Society of Medicine, 105*(3), 111–116. https://doi.org/10.1258/jrsm.2011.110221

Carcelén-García, S., Narros-González, M. J., & Galmes-Cerezo, M. (2023). Digital vulnerability in young people: gender, age and online participation patterns. *International Journal of Adolescence and Youth, 28*(1), 2287115. https://doi.org/10.1080/02673843.2023.2287115

Champion, A. R., Oswald, F., Khera, D., & Pedersen, C. L. (2022). Examining the gendered impacts of technology-facilitated sexual violence: A mixed methods approach. *Archives of Sexual Behavior, 51,* 1607–1624. https://doi.org/10.1007/s10508-021-02226-y

Craig, S. L., Brooks, A. S., Doll, K., Eaton, A. D., McInroy, L. B., & Hui, J. (2023). Processes and manifestations of digital resilience: Video and textual insights from sexual and gender minority youth. *Journal of Adolescent Research, 0*(0). https://doi.org/10.1177/07435584221144958

DeKeseredy, W. S., Schwartz, M. D., Harris, B., Woodlock, D., Nolan, J., & Hall-Sanchez, A. (2019). Technology-facilitated stalking and unwanted sexual messages/images in a college campus community: The role of negative peer support. *SAGE Open, 9*(1), 215824401982823. https://doi.org/10.1177/2158244019828231

Del Prete, A., & Redon Pantoja, S. (2020). Las redes sociales on-line: Espacios de socialización y definición de identidad [On-line social networks: Spaces for socialization and identity definition]. *Psicoperspectivas, 19*(1), 86–96. https://doi.org/10.5027/psicoperspectivas-Vol19-Issue1-fulltext-1834

Derogatis, L. R., & Fitzpatrick, M. (2004). The SCL-90-R, the Brief symptom inventory (BSI), and the BSI-18. In *The use of psychological testing for treatment planning and outcomes assessment: Instruments for adults* (3rd ed., Vol. 3, pp. 1–41). Lawrence Erlbaum Associates Publishers. https://doi.org/10.4324/9781410610614

Donoso, T., Rubio, M. J., & Vilà, R. (2017). Las ciberagresiones en función del género [Cyber-aggressions by gender]. *Revisal de Investigación Educativa, 35*(1), 197–214. https://doi.org/10.6018/rie.35.1.249771

Drechsler, J. (2015). Multiple imputation of multilevel missing data-rigor versus simplicity. *Journal of Educational and Behavioral Statistics, 4*(1), 69–95. http://doi.org/10.3102/1076998614563393

Englander, E. K., & McCoy, M. (2017). Pressured sexting and revenge porn in a sample of Massachusetts adolescents. *International Journal of Technoethics* (IJT), *8*(2), 16–25. https://doi.org/10.4018/IJT.2017070102

Estébanez, I. (2018). *La ciberviolencia hacia las adolescentes en las redes sociales* [Cyberviolence against girls in social networks]. Sevilla, España: Instituto Andaluz de la Mujer. Retrieved from https://goo.gl/hC8s6P

Gámez-Guadix, M., Almendros, C., Calvete, E., & De Santisteban, P. (2018). Persuasion strategies and sexual solicitations and interactions in online sexual grooming of adolescents: Modeling direct and indirect pathways. *Journal of Adolescence, 63*, 11–18. https://doi.org/10.1016/j.adolescence.2017.12.002

Gámez-Guadix, M., Borrajo, E., & Almendros, C. (2016). Risky online behaviors among adolescents: Longitudinal relations among problematic internet use, cyberbullying perpetration, and meeting strangers online. *Journal of Behavioral Addictions, 5*(1), 100–107. https://doi.org/10.1556/2006.5.2016.013

Gámez-Guadix, M., & Íncera, D. (2021). Homophobia is online: Sexual victimization and risks on the internet and mental health among bisexual, homosexual, pansexual, asexual, and queer adolescents. *Computers in Human Behavior, 119.* https://doi.org/10.1016/j.chb.2021.106728

Gámez-Guadix, M., Sorrel, M. A., & Martínez-Bacaicoa, J. (2022). Technology-facilitated sexual violence perpetration and victimization among adolescents: A network analysis. *Sexuality Research & Social Policy, 20.* https://doi.org/10.1007/s13178-022-00775-y

Henry, N., & Powell, A. (2015). Embodied harms: Gender, shame, and technology-facilitated sexual violence. *Violence Against Women, 21*(6), 758–779. https://doi.org/10.1177/1077801215576581

Hillstrom, L. (2018). *The #MeToo Movement.* Retrieved from http://publisher.abc-clio.com/9781440867507

Hsieh, Y. P., Wei, H. S., Lin, Y. S., & Ma, J. K. H. (2023). Understanding the dynamics of unwanted online sexual solicitation among youth in Taiwan: Vulnerability and resilience factors. *Archives of Sexual Behavior, 52*(7), 2799–2810. https://doi.org/10.1007/s10508-023-02719-y

Idoiaga, N., Gil de Montes Echaide, L., Asla, N., & Larrañaga, M. (2020). "La Manada" in the digital sphere: coping with a sexual aggression case through Twitter. *Feminist Media Studies, 20*(7), 926–943. https://doi.org/10.1080/14680777.2019.1643387

Martínez-Bacaicoa, J., Real-Brioso, N., Mateos-Pérez, E., & Gámez-Guadix, M. (2024). The role of gender and sexism in the moral disengagement mechanisms of technology-facilitated sexual violence. *Computers in Human Behavior, 152.* https://doi.org/10.1016/j.chb.2023.108060

Morelli, M., Bianchi, D., Baiocco, R., Pezzuti, L., & Chirumbolo, A. (2016). Sexting, psychological distress and dating violence among adolescents and young adults. *Psicothema, 28*(2), 137–142. https:/doi.org/10.7334/psicothema2015.193

Nadim, M., & Fladmoe, A. (2021). Silencing women? Gender and online harassment. *Social Science Computer Review, 39*(2), 245–258. https://doi.org/10.1177/0894439319865518

Patchin, J. W., & Hinduja, S. (2020). Sextortion among adolescents: Results from a national survey of U.S. youth. *Sexual Abuse, 32*(1), 30–54. https:/doi.org/10.1177/1079063218800469

Pérez-Martínez, V., Sanz-Barbero, B., Ferrer-Cascales, R., Bowes, N., Ayala, A., Sánchez-SanSegundo, M., … Vives-Cases, C. (2021). The role of social support in machismo and acceptance of violence among adolescents in Europe: Lights4violence baseline results. *Journal of Adolescent Health, 68*(5), 922–929. https://doi.org/10.1016/j.jadohealth.2020.09.007

Powell, A., & Henry, N. (2019). Technology-facilitated sexual violence victimization: Results from an online survey of Australian adults. *Journal of Interpersonal Violence, 34*(17), 3637–3665. https://doi.org/10.1177/0886260516672055

Powell, A., Henry, N., & Flynn, A. (2018). Image-based sexual abuse. In W. S. DeKeseredy, & M. Dragiewicz (eds.), *Routledge Handbook of Critical Criminology* (pp. 305–315). New York: Routledge. https://doi.org/10.4324/9781315622040

Reed, E., Salazar, M., Behar, A. I., Agah, N., Silverman, J. G., Minnis, A. M., Rusch, M. L. A., & Raj, A. (2019). Cyber sexual harassment: Prevalence and association with substance use, poor mental health, and STI history among sexually active adolescent girls. *Journal of Adolescence, 75* (1), 53–62 https://doi.org/10.1016/j.adolescence.2019.07.005

Rincón, R. (2019, June 22). El Supremo eleva la condena a La Manada a 15 años: fue una violación múltiple, no un abuso sexual [The Supreme Court raises the sentence of La Manada to 15 years: it was multiple rape, not sexual abuse]. *El País*. https://elpais.com/sociedad/2019/06/21/actualidad/156

Sklenarova, H., Schulz, A., Schuhmann, P., Osterheider, M., & Neutze, J. (2018). Online sexual solicitation by adults and peers—Results from a population based German sample. *Child Abuse & Neglect, 76,* 225–236. https://doi.org/10.1016/j.chiabu.2017.11.005

14

SECTION 2 COMMENTARY

Princesses, Pornography, and Sexual Violence: Understanding the Impact of Teens' Experiences with Sexual Media Content

Stacey J.T. Hust, Rebecca Ortiz, and Jessica Fitts Willoughby

The media are ubiquitous in teens' lives and can include sexual content. The research presented in this section's chapters revealed ways in which teens incorporate some of these sexual media messages into their daily romantic and sexual lives and how media impact can begin as young as early childhood and continue into older adolescence. Ward et al. (Chapter 10) found that, among young women in the United States, greater engagement with Disney princesses during childhood was associated with increased enjoyment of self-sexualization and participation in self-sexualizing behaviors as an older adolescent. Van Ouytsel and colleagues (Chapter 11) found that, for young teens in Belgium, greater internet use was associated with image-based sexting and related sexual abuse behaviors. Densley et al. (Chapter 12) found that viewing sexually explicit media (i.e., pornography) was associated with the production of sexual content (i.e., sexting) for a sample of U.S. adolescents. Martínez-Bacaicoa and coauthors (Chapter 13) found that Spanish adolescents' experiences with technology-facilitated sexual violence were associated with increased anxiety and depression.

Although the research presented in this section investigated the influence of an array of media content, from princess culture to pornography, all four chapters considered adolescents as engaged, active viewers or producers of content instead of passive recipients. For example, Ward and colleagues broadly operationalized Disney princess engagement to include not just watching Disney princess movies but also dressing up as a princess, reading princess books, and playing with princess toys. This operationalization recognizes that the princess phenomenon is about active

DOI: 10.4324/9781032648880-17

engagement with multiple aspects of the princess culture. Furthermore, the results suggest that active incorporation of princess storylines, which often emphasize women's beauty and passivity, into play, dress-up, and role-play as a young child may influence how older adolescent women view their grown-up bodies and roles in romantic and sexual relationships. Similarly, Densley and coauthors found that teens' *consumption* of pornography was associated with their *production* of sexual content via sexting, suggesting that teens may act out some of the sexual behaviors they see (although more research is needed to be sure).

The chapters in this section also included a focus on gender. Previous research has well established that there is a sexual double standard in adolescent romantic and sexual relationships, such that boys are expected to be sexual aggressors and girls are to be sexual gatekeepers (e.g., Hust & Rodgers, 2018). Given these gendered expectations, the chapters in this section considered how a teen's gender may influence their media use and the potential differential gendered effects of the media. Ward and colleagues focused solely on young women, since Disney princesses are specifically marketed to young girls. Densley and colleagues found that while boys were more likely than girls to use pornography, exposure to such content was associated with both boys' and girls' sexting behaviors. Van Ouytsel and colleagues found that boys were more likely than girls to have forwarded a sext without consent, and girls were more likely to experience image-based sexual abuse and adult sexual solicitation. Similarly, Martinez-Bacaicoa and colleagues found that girls were more likely than boys to be victims of all types of technology-facilitated sexual violence (TFSV). In fact, close to half (46%) of the girls in the study had experienced TFSV.

Taken together, these chapters reveal that media help create an environment in which young girls are at greater risk of sexual violence than boys, specifically online. Although boys are not immune, the burden of victimization is largely felt among young girls, and therefore, these gender differences must be acknowledged. Parents and schools must adopt educational efforts (e.g., media literacy) that empower young people to critically evaluate sexual media messages and adopt internet safety practices, as well as teach, especially young boys, about not engaging in abusive online and digital behaviors. Parents, schools, religious organizations, and sociocultural environments all play roles in shaping youths' romantic and sexual beliefs and behaviors, and media scholars draw on theories such as ecological systems theory (Brofenbrenner, 1992), social cognitive theory (Bandura, 2001; Bussey & Bandura, 1999), and the integrated model of behavioral prediction (Fishbein, 2009) to argue that media contribute uniquely to such beliefs, especially in the absence of protective factors (e.g., parental mediation or access to media literacy). Therefore, it is imperative in this work to recognize the multiple systems at play.

Victims of sexual violence, however, cannot and should not be expected to protect themselves online as a first line of defense. Instead, policies and legislation must reduce and address all aspects of TFSV victimization and perpetration. Although the research in these chapters specifically looked at boys and girls or young women, other research has found that adolescents with historically marginalized identities, such as racial, ethnic, gender, and/or sexual minority youth, can be at increased risk of experiencing sexual violence (e.g., Sheats et al., 2018; Williams & Gutierrez, 2021) and therefore also deserve special consideration. Additionally, Martinez-Bacaicoa and colleagues found that experiences with TFSV were associated with increased anxiety and depression, revealing the potential harmful effects of these experiences.

These studies further our understanding of mediated sexual violence by broadening the definition to include nonconsensual behaviors within a mobile environment and online perpetration of sexual violence. The results suggest that studies of and efforts to address sexual violence should consider behaviors that occur both online and offline. However, unlike the TFSV behaviors that Martinez-Bacaicoa and colleagues discuss, it is unclear how consensual image-based sexting fits within the existing definitions of romantic and sexual behavior and sexual violence. As Van Ouytsel and colleagues point out, among some adolescents, sexting is a natural developmental step that may allow teens to explore sexual relationships without the same physical consequences as offline sexual activity. Yet they also differentiated consensual image-based sexting from nonconsensual image-based sexual abuse. Other scholars, however, may argue that any image-based sexting by a minor should be considered child pornography. These results suggest that media scholars may have a unique opportunity to help inform policies and practices related to image-based sexting. Scholars could help define what consensual sexting looks like among adolescents and could help establish whether image-based sexting should be included in such a definition.

Although these studies each uniquely contribute to the field, they are not without limitations. Some studies in this section examined gender as binary (e.g., boy/girl). This leaves unanswered questions about how nonbinary or gender-fluid individuals may have attended to these media and how sexual media content may affect them differently. Additionally, these studies did not account for differences based on sexual orientation. For example, LGBTQ+ youths may experience some types of TFSV, such as gender-based violence and sexual-orientation-based violence, more than their heterosexual counterparts (Srivastava et al., 2022). Future studies should specifically explore the effects of engaging in and attending to sexual media content among LGBTQ+ populations. With the exception of Martinez-Bacaicoa and colleagues' chapter, each of the chapters was based on cross-sectional surveys. Additional longitudinal and experimental research is needed to better understand how and why sexual media affect adolescents. In-depth qualitative research could also help inform our understanding of how adolescents make sense of sexual media and the processes through which they internalize sexual media messages. See Chapters 1 and 2 for more discussion on this.

Despite these limitations, these chapters extend existing research and provide a strong foundation from which the field can continue to build investigations into the effects of sexual media content. As Ward and colleagues identified, childhood engagement with princess-related media was associated with young women's body beliefs in older adolescents. Such beliefs could result in many negative health behaviors, which should be further investigated. Martinez-Bacaicoa and colleagues identified that experiences with TFSV were associated with anxiety and depression. Overall, the results provide evidence that sexual content on traditional and digital media may be associated with youths' physical and mental health and should be considered a pressing concern for scholars and health communication practitioners alike. These studies also suggest that future research must take care to precisely and carefully operationalize media exposure and to account for the myriad ways in which adolescents engage with and internalize the media messages to which they attend.

References

Bandura, A. (2001). Social cognitive theory of mass communication. *Media Psychology*, *3*(3), 265–299. https://doi.org/10.1207/s1532785Xmep0303_03

Bronfenbrenner, U. (1992). Ecological systems theory. In R. Vasta (ed.), *Six theories of child development: Revised formulations and current issues*(pp. 187–249). Jessica Kingsley Publishers.

Bussey, K., & Bandura, A. (1999). Social cognitive theory of gender development and differentiation. *Psychological Review*, *106*(4), 676–713. https://doi.org/10.1037/0033-295X.106.4.676

Fishbein, M. (2009). An integrative model for behavioral prediction and its application to health promotion. In R. J. DiClemente, R. A. Crosby, & M. C. Kegler (Eds.), *Emerging theories in health promotion practice and research* (2nd ed., pp. 215–234). Jossey-Bass/Wiley.

Hust, S. J. T. & Rodgers, K. B. (2018). *Scripting adolescent romance: Adolescents talk about romantic relationships and media's sexual scripts*. Mediated Youth Series, Peter Lang Publishing.

Sheats, K. J., Irving, S. M., Mercy, J. A., Simon, T. R., Crosby, A. E., Ford, D. C., Merrick, M. T., Annor, F. B., & Morgan, R. E. (2018). Violence-related disparities experienced by black youth and young adults: Opportunities for prevention. *American Journal of Preventive Medicine, 55*(4), 462–469. https://doi.org/10.1016/j.amepre.2018.05.017

Srivastava, A., Rusow, J., Schrager, S. M., Stephenson, R., & Goldbach, J. T. (2022). Digital sexual violence and suicide risk in a national sample of sexual minority adolescents. *Journal of Interpersonal Violence, 38*(3–4), 4443–4458. https://doi.org/10.1177/08862605221116317

Williams, R. D., & Gutierrez, A. (2021). Increased likelihood of forced sexual intercourse, sexual violence, and sexual dating violence victimization among sexual minority youth. *Journal of Community Health, 47*(2), 193–200. https://doi.org/10.1007/s10900-021-01033-9

SECTION 3

Adolescents as Engagers and Creators

Opportunities for Media Education and Advocacy

15

SECTION 3 INTRODUCTION

Adolescents as Engagers and Creators: Opportunities for Media Education and Advocacy

Jessica Fitts Willoughby

Teens frequently engage with media, including in the creation of media (e.g., Guerrero-Pico et al., 2019). Research has highlighted the benefits of the co-production of digital sexual health services, made in partnership with adolescents (Bennett et al., 2023), and the benefits of furthering the involvement of young people in intervention and campaign development (e.g., Martin et al., 2020; Ortiz & Shafer, 2018). Bennett et al. (2023) concluded in their review of digital interventions that the design of digital interventions would benefit from reflecting the needs of adolescents and creating interventions that adolescents feel comfortable using, while also addressing potential barriers. Specifically, they state that the emphasis on adolescents' perspectives is "vital to unleash the full potential of digital technology in this domain" (p. 2).

Media have often been used successfully for health promotion efforts in the areas of sexual and reproductive health (e.g., Wadham et al., 2019). In a systematic review that examined 25 studies that used digital sexual health interventions for people ages 13–24, Wadham et al. (2019) found success of some interventions, including at influencing knowledge related to HIV and STI prevention and sexual health knowledge, as well as effects related to condom-use intentions. However, they noted that digital interventions need to have high-quality, evidence-based content with which young people can engage.

This involvement of young people in the creation of content and the various ways in which they can engage with content differ significantly from generations past. The internet has brought with it a host of resources, including technology-based interventions for health promotion efforts and

DOI: 10.4324/9781032648880-19

the ability for teens to seek out sexual health information, including via mobile devices (e.g., Willoughby, 2015; Willoughby & Muldrow, 2017). However, even with the plethora of resources literally at their fingertips, or maybe because of them, teens report that they have struggled to identify accurate and relevant sexual health information (e.g., Farrugia et al., 2021). Past work has found that how adolescents and young adults make sense of media content can impact their interpretations of content (e.g., Hust et al., 2019; Smith & Ortiz, 2023; Willoughby et al., 2022; Willoughby et al., 2024). Media literacy, which is one's ability to access, analyze, create, and act using various communication (National Association for Media Literacy Education, 2024), can also impact how media affects young people. In these next four chapters, the authors will provide you with some specific examples of opportunities related to media in the areas of sexual health promotion, including how adolescents engage with and create content as well as how their understanding of such content can influence sexual health-related outcomes.

In Chapter 16, Dodson and Scull describe the media literacy program *Media Aware* as a case study and describe the results of multiple randomized controlled trials testing iterations of *Media Aware* delivered to adolescents across developmental age ranges. They provide examples of how media literacy can have a positive impact on attitudes and behaviors and highlight key takeaways from their findings. Additionally, they showcase how media literacy education can be useful as a form of sexual health education, providing adolescents with information pertinent for healthy sexual relationships.

Young people often seek out sexual health information online, although they do not often have trust in the information they may find (Farrugia et al., 2021). In Chapter 17, Zelaya and colleagues provide insights into the sexual health-related information seeking of adolescents and their understanding of content in retrospective reports about what young adults think would have been helpful information to have in digital sexual health resources. Based on data drawn from a sample of 300 18- to 24-year-olds from the United States, they used thematic analysis to examine young adults' responses to an open-ended question in which participants were asked to think back to their younger years and identify the sexuality and sexual health information they wish they had access to online during that time.

In Chapter 18, Riggs and colleagues examine whether there may be sexual health education benefits to viewing even negative portrayals in mass media, such as those related to sexual violence. Riggs and colleagues use an experiment and qualitative insights gathered among 13- to 17-year-olds in the United States to examine how teens responded to media content that presented supportive and unsupportive sexual assault victimization narratives on their self-efficacy related to sharing the story in comparison to sharing a control condition story.

In Chapter 19, Willoughby and colleagues continue the examination of mass media and digital media as areas in which teens may learn sexual health information to see how teens are further communicating their attitudes and opinions related to sexual and reproductive health and may be advocating for themselves and others. The authors examine how 18- to 20-year-olds in the United States, Australia, and the United Kingdom are sharing their concerns related to contraceptive access, STI testing and prevention, menstrual product access and abortion rights, and whether those online behaviors are associated with attending rallies and demonstrations.

Taken together, section three of this text highlights areas in which we see promise for media to serve young people as a form of health communication and for young people to use their voices, as creators and engagers with media, to influence adolescent sexual and reproductive health.

References

Bennett, C., Musa, M. K., Carrier, J., Edwards, D., Gillen, E., Sydor, A., ... & Kelly, D. (2023). The barriers and facilitators to young people's engagement with bidirectional digital sexual health interventions: A mixed methods systematic review. *BMC Digital Health*, 1(1), 30. https://doi.org/10.1186/s44247-023-00030-3

Farrugia, A., Waling, A., Pienaar, K., & Fraser, S. (2021). The "be all and end all"? Young people, online sexual health information, science and skepticism. *Qualitative Health Research*, 31(11), 2097–2110. https://doi.org/10.1177/10497323211003543

Guerrero-Pico, M., Masanet, M. J., & Scolari, C. A. (2019). Toward a typology of young produsers: Teenagers' transmedia skills, media production, and narrative and aesthetic appreciation. *New Media & Society*, 21(2), 336–353. https://doi.org/10.1177/1461444818796470

Hust, S. J., Rodgers, K. B., Cameron, N., & Li, J. (2019). Viewers' perceptions of objectified images of women in alcohol advertisements and their intentions to intervene in alcohol-facilitated sexual assault situations. *Journal of Health Communication*, 24(3), 328–338. https://doi.org/10.1080/10810730.2019.1604911

Martin, P., Cousin, L., Gottot, S., Bourmaud, A., de La Rochebrochard, E., & Alberti, C. (2020). Participatory interventions for sexual health promotion for adolescents and young adults on the internet: Systematic review. *Journal of Medical Internet Research*, 22(7), e15378. https://doi.org/10.2196/15378

National Association for Media Literacy Education. (2024). *What is media literacy?* https://namle.org/resources/media-literacy-defined/

Ortiz, R. R., & Shafer, A. (2018). Unblurring the lines of sexual consent with a college student-driven sexual consent education campaign. *Journal of American College Health*, 66(6), 450–456. https://doi.org/10.1080/07448481.2018.1431902

Smith, A. M., & Ortiz, R. R. (2023). How college students interpret and use social media as a potential source of sexual consent communication. *Social Media + Society, 9*(3). https://doi.org/10.1177/20563051221147332

Wadham, E., Green, C., Debattista, J., Somerset, S., & Sav, A. (2019). New digital media interventions for sexual health promotion among young people: A systematic review. *Sexual Health, 16*(2), 101–123. https://doi.org/10.1071/SH18127

Willoughby, J. F. (2015). BrdsNBz: Sexually experienced teens more likely to use sexual health text message service. *Health Education & Behavior, 42*(6), 752–758. https://doi.org/10.1177/1090198115577377

Willoughby, J. F., Hust, S.J.T., Couto, L., Li, J., Kang, S., Nickerson, C. G., ... & Tlachi-Munoz, S. (2024). The impact of sexual scripts in brand-generated cannabis social media posts on sex-related cannabis expectancies: Does body appreciation moderate effects? *Drug and Alcohol Review, 43*(1), 122–131. https://doi.org/10.1111/dar.13642

Willoughby, J. F., Hust, S.J.T., Li, J., & Couto, L. (2022). Social media, marijuana and sex: An exploratory study of adolescents' intentions to use and college students' use of marijuana. *The Journal of Sex Research, 59*(1), 85–97. https://doi.org/10.1080/00224499.2020.1827217

Willoughby, J. F., & Muldrow, A. (2017). SMS for sexual health: A comparison of service types and recommendations for sexual health text message service providers. *Health Education Journal, 76*(2), 231–243. https://doi.org/10.1177/0017896916661373

16

MEDIA LITERACY EDUCATION FOR COMPREHENSIVE SEXUAL HEALTH PROMOTION

Christina V. Dodson and Tracy M. Scull

Media literacy is often defined as "the ability to access, analyze, evaluate, create, and act using all forms of communication" (National Association for Media Literacy Education, 2024). Media literacy is a broad concept, but at its core is the idea that a media literate individual is an informed and active media consumer and producer, equipped to navigate media with a critical awareness (see Dodson et al., 2024). With that said, we think that Dr. Jane D. Brown said it best in describing her favorite simple definition, "we're teaching adolescents how to read 'Baywatch' as well as 'Beowulf'" (Brown, 2006). Many years later, this definition held true, but, in today's digital environment, we're also teaching adolescents to read "TikTok" as well as "Twelfth Night."

Media are an important part of sexual socialization (Scull & Malik, 2019; Ward, 2003; Ward et al., 2019; Wright, 2009). However, media often present inaccurate, unrealistic, and unhealthy information about sex (e.g., Dillman Carpentier et al., 2017), and exposure to sexual content in both pornography (Peter & Valkenburg, 2016) and mainstream/entertainment media (Coyne et al., 2019) predicts adolescents' sexual cognitions and behaviors. Parental media restriction can have a protective effect on adolescent sexual health outcomes (Collier et al., 2016); however, it is imperative that adolescents are media literate so they can critically navigate the sexual media content that they will inevitably encounter.

Media literacy can be taught through media literacy education (MLE). Although its origins date back further, the concept of MLE took root in the United States as a field of study starting in the 1950s focusing on films and propaganda (Hobbs & Jensen, 2009). By the early 2000s, MLE was

DOI: 10.4324/9781032648880-20

an established field, but in its nascency as an approach to health education and was just being proposed as a promising approach to *sexual* health education (e.g., Brown, 2006). Since then, MLE for health education has experienced exciting growth, and meta-analyses have established that MLE is effective in improving a variety of health outcomes including those related to substance use, violence, body image, and sexual health (Jeong et al., 2012; Vahedi et al., 2018; Xie et al., 2019).

Media literacy education for adolescent sexual health promotion

There are multiple perspectives and approaches regarding MLE and sexual health education in the United States, and, like all researchers, our work is shaped, in part, by our personal experiences and viewpoints. As both researchers and parents of tweens and teens, we are dedicated to empowering youth to make informed sexual choices and leverage media to enhance sexual well-being. We advocate for evidence-based, medically-accurate, inclusive, and comprehensive sexual health education, and feel that media literacy is an essential life skill. More than a decade ago, we were connected by Dr. Jane D. Brown and, inspired by her work, began our own research developing and evaluating MLE programs with these goals in mind. Guided by theory, our work has explored MLE's impact on adolescents' media- and sexual health-related cognitions and behaviors.

Theoretical frameworks

There are multiple theories valuable in guiding MLE research. Our work has been informed by theories of media effects and health behavior. Theories of media message processing can be useful in identifying variables that either amplify or attenuate the influence of media exposure on health. For example, the Message Interpretation Process model posits that critical media attitudes (e.g., perceived realism of media messages) mediate the impact of media exposure on health behaviors (Austin & Johnson, 1997), and dual process theories of persuasion (e.g., Chaiken & Trope, 1999; Petty & Cacioppo, 1986) have shown that the persuasiveness of a media message is impacted, in part, by the scrutiny with which the message is processed. Theories of health behavior change can guide researchers in exploring how MLE impacts predictors of health cognitions and, ultimately, behaviors. For example, the Theory of Planned Behavior (Ajzen, 1991) posits that attitudes, normative beliefs, and self-efficacy predict sexual intentions which, in turn, predict behavior.

Critical media attitudes and media message processing skills

Critical media attitudes reflect a level of distrust or disbelief in what is being conveyed in media and are thought to encourage more careful processing of media messages (see Baams et al., 2015; Dodson et al., 2024). Two important critical media attitudes related to sexual media messages are perceived realism and media skepticism. Perceived realism is the extent to which one judges media content to be similar to the real world (Busselle & Greenberg, 2000), and media skepticism pertains to one's level of mistrust toward the media (Tsfati, 2003). Critical media attitudes have been found to inversely predict intentions to engage in sexual activity (Scull, Malik, & Kupersmidt, 2018) and attenuate the negative impact of sexual media exposure on health-related outcomes, including engaging in condomless sex (Wright et al., 2022) and acceptance of rape myths (Evans-Paulson et al., 2023).

Given adolescents' oftentimes limited sexual experiences, they may be more prone to accepting sexual media portrayals as reflecting reality, which can lead them to think teen sex is more normative than it is in reality (Coyne et al., 2019). This can be especially harmful when risky sexual behaviors are depicted in media without consequence; this can lead to adolescents underestimating the consequences of risky sexual behaviors in real life (see Scull & Malik, 2019; Ward et al., 2016). Similarly, adolescents' trust in and identification with certain celebrities and social media influencers may make them especially vulnerable to persuasion and influence from these sources (Lou & Kim, 2019; Schouten et al., 2021). By decreasing perceived realism and increasing skepticism, MLE can encourage adolescents to question sexual media messages rather than simply trusting and accepting them as factual (see Dodson et al., 2024). More careful scrutiny of sexual media messages can encourage the rejection of messages promoting unhealthy sexual beliefs and behaviors. For example, MLE can teach students to reflect on the overt and implied messages being conveyed in sexual media messages about gender, romantic relationships, and sex, and carefully evaluate the accuracy and completeness of sexual media messages (Scull et al., 2022; Scull, Kupersmidt, Malik, & Keefe, 2018; Scull, Kupersmidt, Malik, & Morgan-Lopez, 2018). MLE can also teach students to reflect on the impact of sexual media messages on themselves, their peers, and society (Dodson et al., 2024). This enhanced message processing encourages adolescents to think critically about sexual media messages as opposed to being passively influenced by them.

Sexual health knowledge and cognitions

In addition to enhancing students' critical media attitudes and media message processing skills, it is important that MLE for sexual health education also impacts students' sexual health knowledge and beliefs (see Dodson et al., 2024). For example, as adolescents learn media literacy skills, they may compare the information in media with their own sexual health knowledge to determine if the information in the message is accurate. Imagine a student is considering getting a long-acting reversible contraceptive, like an intrauterine device (IUD), for birth control. They start seeing social media posts in which people are talking about failure rates (e.g., "baby was born with the IUD in their hand"). If they are media literate and analyze these messages to evaluate their accuracy, they likely compare the message to their existing knowledge about IUD efficacy. If they believe that IUDs are *not* effective in preventing pregnancy or are not sure, they are likely to determine that the social media posts are accurate, and they may be dissuaded from getting an IUD. However, if they have knowledge that IUDs are 99% effective in preventing pregnancy (United States Food and Drug Administration, 2023), they are more likely to reject the accuracy of the posts.

Sexual health cognitions, such as normative beliefs, attitudes, and self-efficacy, are established predictors of sexual health intentions and behaviors (Buhi & Goodson, 2007; Sheeran et al., 2016) and, therefore, variables of importance in MLE for sexual health promotion. Media often over-emphasize sexual behaviors (e.g., portraying teen sex and risky sexual behaviors as commonplace; Ward, 2003). Sexual media exposure is associated with adolescents' more permissive attitudes about sex and normative beliefs regarding peer sexual activity (Coyne et al., 2019). Therefore, by correcting adolescents' inaccurate normative beliefs about the prevalence of teen sex and risky sexual activity, students are less likely to engage in these activities. In addition, media messages have been found to promote gender roles and sexual stereotypes, normalize unhealthy relationships, and perpetuate rape myths (Hedrick, 2021; Ward & Grower, 2020). Redressing these beliefs, which are associated with sexual and relationship violence (Reyes et al., 2016; Yapp & Quayle, 2018), can protect against adolescents engaging in these harmful behaviors. Sexual media messages often omit information about sexual health communication (i.e., talking with parents, medical professionals, and partners about sexual health) and contraception/protection (Dillman Carpentier et al., 2017). If adolescents are turning to media for sex education, they will likely not receive accurate, or possibly any, information about these topics. MLE can fill this gap by providing sexual health information that is often missing from media messages, which has been found to improve sexual health.

Case study: *Media Aware* programs

Our research team has developed and evaluated a series of MLE programs for comprehensive sexual health education – *Media Aware*.

These programs are designed to impact adolescents' media-related outcomes (i.e., critical media attitudes; critical media message processing) and health-related outcomes (i.e., sexual health knowledge; sexual health cognitions) with the ultimate goal of empowering adolescents to make informed and healthy sexual decisions. They include a teacher-led program for younger adolescents that can be taught across ten 50-minute class periods (*Media Aware* for Middle School), a web-based program for older adolescents that can be completed across four class periods (*Media Aware* for High School), and a self-paced online program for young adults ages 18-22 that can be completed on a phone, tablet, or computer at a student's own pace (*Media Aware* for Young Adults).

Program content

The *Media Aware* programs are developmentally-appropriate comprehensive sexual health education programs designed to meet several state and national sexual health education guidelines. Although the programs differ in length and format, all of the programs are designed to impact health outcomes by enhancing critical media analysis. Throughout the program, students watch and listen to a variety of relevant media examples from television, movies, music, YouTube, social media, and more. They learn how to critically analyze and evaluate sexual media messages guided by key media literacy questions (e.g., What are the goals of this message? Who is benefiting from this message and who is potentially being harmed?). In addition to enhancing media literacy skills, the analysis and evaluation of sexual media messages serve as a platform to teach medically-accurate sexual and relationship health information. Sexual health topics covered in the program include: gender role stereotypes; healthy and unhealthy relationships; intimate partner violence; sexual violence; bystander intervention; substance use and sex; STI transmission, prevention and treatment; pregnancy prevention including FDA-approved methods of contraception; and, effective sexual health communication. Interactive activities guide the students in comparing medically-accurate health information to the information being communicated in media to evaluate the realism, accuracy, and completeness of media messages (for additional program details see mediaawareprograms.com and mediaawarecollegeprograms.com).

Program evaluations

The efficacy of the *Media Aware* programs has been assessed through U.S.-based randomized control trials funded by the National Institutes of Health to examine the impact of the programs on short-term outcomes among middle school students (7th and 8th grade classes; Scull, Kupersmidt,

Malik, & Morgan-Lopez, 2018), high school students (9th and 10th grade classes; Scull et al., 2022), and young adults attending community college (students 18 and 19 years of age; Scull, Kupersmidt, Malik, & Keefe, 2018). The middle school and high school studies employed a pretest–posttest design (i.e., 1–2 weeks between pretest and posttest) with an active control (i.e., between pretest and posttest students in the control condition received health education content that did not include sexual health nor MLE), and the young adult study employed a pretest-posttest design (i.e., 4 weeks between pretest and posttest) with a wait-list control (i.e., students did not receive any health or MLE between pretest and posttest). Study approval was obtained from the innovation Research & Training Internal Review Board and informed consent was obtained for all participants in these studies. The findings from these rigorous evaluations demonstrate the programs' success in influencing both media-related and sexual health-related outcomes[1] (see Table 16.1) and illuminate directions for program refinement, additional program development, and implementation research. Taken together, several key takeaways for MLE for sexual health education have emerged from this research.

Takeaway #1: MLE can positively impact cognitions and skills that predict sexual health behaviors and attenuate the potentially harmful impact of media on sexual health

The *Media Aware* programs were found to enhance critical media attitudes and media message processing skills in addition to impacting sexual health knowledge and cognitions related to sexual health. Although several traditional (i.e., not MLE) evidence-based sexual health education programs have been found to impact sexual health knowledge and cognitions, they rarely teach students how to effectively navigate and think critically about sexual media messages. Our evaluations of *Media Aware* revealed that, compared to the control conditions, the middle school and young adult programs enhanced students' skepticism of sexually-themed media messages and the high school program resulted in students perceiving sexually-themed media messages as less realistic. Our evaluations of the middle and high school programs also revealed that these programs enhanced students' ability to critically analyze or deconstruct media messages. This research suggests that a MLE approach can enhance adolescent health by impacting cognitive predictors of sexual health behaviors (e.g., normative beliefs, attitudes, self-efficacy) *and* media-related cognitions and skills that serve as protective factors against the potentially negative effects of sexual media exposure on adolescent sexual health outcomes (e.g., perceived media realism, media skepticism, critical media message processing). This provides evidence that

TABLE 16.1 *Media Aware* program primary evaluations select findings

Outcome	Sample Item	Sample Citation	Program MS	HS	YA
Critical Media Attitudes and Media Message Processing Skills					
Perceived media realism*	Teens in the media are as sexually active as average teens. (strongly disagree – strongly agree)	(adapted from Austin & Johnson, 1997)	*ns*	X	*ns*
Media skepticism*	Media are dishonest about what happens if people have sex. (strongly disagree – strongly agree)	(Scull, Kupersmidt, Malik, & Morgan-Lopez, 2018)	X	*ns*	X (men)
Media deconstruction skills**	1) Tell us about the advertisement in the space below (the more detail the better). 2) How are advertisers trying to get someone to buy this product? 3) Is there anything missing from the ad?	(Kupersmidt et al., 2010; Scull et al., 2014)	X	X	*ns*
Sexual Health Knowledge, Cognitions, and Behaviors					
Sexual health knowledge	How can someone get a sexually transmitted infection? Select all that apply. (oral sex; genital-to-genital contact; vagina sex)	(Scull et al., 2022)	X	X	X
Normative beliefs/ acceptance of unhealthy beliefs					
Adolescent sexual activity	What percentage of people your age are having sex?	(Scull et al., 2022)	*ns*	X (girls)	X

(Continued)

TABLE 16.1 (Continued)

Outcome	Sample Item	Sample Citation	Program		
			MS	HS	YA
Risky sexual activity	What percentage of people my age are having sex with casual partners?	(Scull et al., 2022)	N/A	X	X
Dating violence acceptance*	It is OK for people to hit their girlfriend/boyfriend if they did something to make them mad. (strongly disagree – strongly agree)	(adapted from Foshee et al., 2005)	X	X (boys)	N/A
Strict gender role acceptance*	Men should be smarter than their girlfriends. (strongly disagree – strongly agree)	(adapted from Foshee et al., 2005)	X	ns	N/A
Rape myth acceptance*	If a girl doesn't say no, she can't claim rape. (strongly disagree – strongly agree)	(adapted from McMahon & Farmer, 2011)	N/A	ns	X
Attitudes					
Sexual health communication*	Before deciding to have sex, I believe that teens should talk with their parent(s) or another trusted adult. (strongly disagree – strongly agree)	(adapted from Halpern-Felsher et al., 2004)	X	N/A	ns
Contraception/protection use*	Condoms should always be used if a person has casual sex. (strongly disagree – strongly agree)	(adapted from Basen-Engquist et al., 1999)	X	N/A	X
Self-efficacy					
Sexual health communication*	I can talk to any potential partner to make him/her understand why we should use condoms or other contraception. (strongly disagree – strongly agree)	(Scull, Kupersmidt, Malik, & Keefe, 2018)	X	ns	X
Contraception/protection use*	I can use a dental dam correctly or explain to my partner how to use a dental dam correctly. (strongly disagree – strongly agree)	(Scull, Kupersmidt, Malik, & Keefe, 2018)	X	ns	X

	Item	Source	MS	HS	YA
Intentions					
Sexual health communication*	Before deciding to have sex, how likely would you be to talk with your parents or another trusted adult about sexual health? (not at all likely – extremely likely)	(adapted from Halpern-Felsher et al., 2004)	X	ns	ns
Contraception/protection use*	If you were to decide to have oral sex in the next six months, how likely would you be to use a condom or dental dam? (not at all likely – very likely)	(Scull, Kupersmidt, Malik, & Keefe, 2018)	X	ns	X (women)
Willingness to have unprotected sex*	Suppose your boyfriend/girlfriend wanted to have sex, but neither of you have protection. How willing would you be to have sex anyway? (not at all willing – very willing)	(adapted from Gibbons et al., 1998; Myklestad & Rise, 2007)	N/A	ns	X
Behaviors					
Risky sexual behaviors	In the past month, how many times have you had sex with someone of unknown STI status?	(adapted from Turchik & Garske, 2008)	N/A	N/A	X
Sexual health communication (with parent)*	How often do you talk with a parent or another trusted adult about sexual health? (Never – Often)	(adapted from Scull et al., 2014)	ns	X (girls)	ns

MS = *Media Aware* for Middle School; HS = *Media Aware* for High School; YA = *Media Aware* for Young Adults; *ns* = not significant; N/A = *variable was not part of the evaluation.*

* Items measured using Likert-type scales.

** Media deconstruction is a performance-based measure used to assess media analysis skills. Students view a sexual media message (e.g., an advertisement that uses sexual themes to promote alcohol) and respond to open ended questions about the message. These responses are then coded by researchers to evaluate the students' media analysis skills.

MLE is an effective approach to sexual health education that goes beyond traditional methods to enhance media-related attitudes and skills that can reduce the impact of unhealthy media messages on sexual behavior.

This research also suggests that the process of critical media analysis and evaluation taught in MLE is effective in enhancing students' critical media attitudes and media message processing skills. Although more research is needed, it is possible that through the building of media literacy skills and the acquisition of accurate sexual health information, adolescents begin to apply their sexual health knowledge when they analyze sexual media messages enabling them to counterargue inaccuracies in sexual media content. This, in turn, may redress inaccurate normative beliefs and misinformation about sex and relationships that are often perpetuated in media messages.

Takeaway #2: MLE can positively impact adolescents' sexual health behaviors

Our research has established that MLE can impact sexual behaviors as well as behavioral intentions and willingness, which are established predictors of behavior. Specifically, the middle school program increased students' intentions to engage in communication about sexual health with medical professionals and partners and resulted in increased intentions for using contraception/protection if they were to engage in sexual activity. Our evaluation of the *Media Aware* for high school program indicated the program resulted in behavior change; specifically, the program resulted in girls' reporting more frequent sexual health communication with their parents. Although immediate changes in sexual behavior were not anticipated, particularly among younger adolescents, many of whom are not sexually active, noteworthy short-term changes in young adults' sexual behaviors were observed. Specifically, a reduction in risky sexual behaviors was seen among young adults ages 18 and 19 including reporting that they engaged in fewer instances of sexual activity with someone who has not been tested for STIs or whose STI status is unknown and, for men, fewer instances of sexual activity with a casual partner and fewer instances of using drugs or alcohol before a sexual encounter. This suggests that MLE holds promise for impacting adolescents' emerging sexual behaviors and improving sexual health.

Takeaway #3: MLE as a form of sexual health education is highly acceptable to adolescents

The evaluations of the *Media Aware* programs assessed student feedback on the program content. Across all three programs, students reported having positive experiences using the programs. Specifically, they found the lessons interesting, reported they learned a lot from the lessons, were glad they learned the lessons, and would recommend the program to a friend or thought it was a good program for other adolescents. It is possible that students think favorably of MLE for sexual health education because it uses popular media examples that they find relevant and engaging. It is also possible that adolescents find MLE engaging because they are avid media consumers and producers and MLE provides them with important skills that they can directly apply to their media consumption and media production choices. Although MLE programs vary greatly and there is an opportunity for future research to explore what aspects of MLE appeal most to students and how these elements affect the efficacy of MLE programs, our program evaluations provide consistent evidence that students find MLE to be an acceptable approach to sexual health education.

Takeaway #4: MLE shows promise for comprehensive sexual health education across developmental stages and across multiple pedagogical formats

Our research revealed that MLE can effectively enhance adolescent media- and sexual health-related outcomes as early as 7th grade and into early adulthood (ages 18 and 19). However, research is needed to better understand how MLE can progressively build adolescents' media literacy and sexual decision-making skills throughout adolescence to impact sexual health behaviors as they emerge. This highlights the importance of employing a developmental framework when developing and implementing MLE for sexual health promotion, which takes into consideration changes in adolescent sexual development, cognitive maturity, and media usage and processing that occur during adolescence. MLE programs are often developed to be taught via in-person classroom settings, yet our research revealed that MLE for sexual health promotion can be effectively delivered via a web-based self-paced format. Even though future research is needed to compare program effects across various pedagogical formats, our research highlights the promise of web-based MLE for sexual health promotion.

Discussion

Media are an integral part of adolescents' lives and sexual socialization. It is unrealistic to think that adolescents could (or should) be "protected" from all sexual media content. It is developmentally appropriate for adolescents to seek information about sex, and media can be used to promote sexual health (e.g., Gabarron & Wynn, 2016). Furthermore, with the inconsistency of school-based sexual health education in the United States (Guttmacher Institute, 2023), adolescents look to media to fill the gaps in their knowledge. Despite this, adolescents receive little, if any, guidance on how to navigate or think critically about sexual media messages. Our research establishes that MLE is an effective approach to sexual health education across adolescence that can impact young people's ability to think critically about sexual media messages and make healthier sexual decisions. Media effects research has illuminated important variables that can attenuate the potentially harmful impact of sexual media messages on sexual decision-making (e.g., perceived realism; skepticism; and media message processing). MLE provides an exciting opportunity to apply those learnings to better understand how those media-related cognitions and skills can be taught to adolescents to impact how they process the media messages they consume and produce each day and, ultimately, empower them to make informed and healthy sexual decisions.

Implications for researchers

There is a strong and growing evidence base for leveraging MLE for health promotion. There are also many unanswered questions in the field and limitations to current MLE research, including our own work. It is promising that our evaluations of MLE programs for sexual health promotion have shown short-term behavioral change, and there is also a need for longitudinal work to explore the impact of MLE programs on emerging sexual and media behaviors over time. In addition, there is a need to better understand the mechanisms through which MLE impacts adolescent sexual health outcomes. For example, we are currently conducting research to better understand how media-related (e.g., realism; skepticism) and health-related (e.g., normative beliefs) constructs influenced by MLE potentially moderate the relationship between adolescent sexual media exposure and sexual behaviors. Understanding how media literacy skills are applied when navigating media at home and other non-academic settings warrants attention, as does research on the implementation of MLE for sexual health education in schools. The field of MLE for health promotion is rapidly expanding, offering opportunities for researchers to explore underlying mechanisms and develop frameworks to explain and refine the measurement of MLE constructs.

Implications for practitioners

School-based comprehensive sexual health education faces considerable challenges. Not all schools require that sexual health education be taught, and, when it is taught, the content and quality vary by state, district, school, and teacher (see SIECUS, 2024). Sometimes with little or no training in sexual health education, teachers (and oftentimes, coaches) are frequently uncomfortable teaching this content. MLE offers a promising solution. Our work has revealed that teachers found using MLE to be an easier avenue to teaching sexual health than traditional (non-MLE) curricula (Scull, Kupersmidt, Malik, & Morgan-Lopez, 2018), and our research suggests that students respond favorably to MLE for sexual health education (Scull et al., 2022; Scull, Kupersmidt, Malik, & Keefe, 2018; Scull, Kupersmidt, Malik, & Morgan-Lopez, 2018). Our research shows promise for the use of MLE in different pedagogical formats thus giving school districts options for implementation including teacher-led MLE, which can be ideal for schools that prioritize project- and group-based learning. A web-based approach has advantages for schools including standardization of content across classes, the ability to update the program for medical accuracy, and the ability for schools to deliver programming to large numbers of students across various educational settings (e.g., in-person classrooms, fully remote learning environment, homeschool settings). We also acknowledge that some schools are prohibited from teaching certain content due to the political and cultural climate. Web-based programming can provide the flexibility for districts and schools to customize content to meet the needs of their students within political constraints, as well as the ability for parents to easily review curriculum content. Regardless of curriculum format, there is a need for teachers to have access to high-quality professional development to prepare them to effectively teach comprehensive sexual health education and MLE.

Looking ahead: The future of MLE for comprehensive sexual health promotion

Media can influence all aspects of our lives in both positive and harmful ways, and sexual health is not an exception. It is inevitable that technology will continue to evolve and advance, and new media technologies will continue to influence adolescents' sexual health. It is imperative that young people, as media consumers and producers, are equipped to critically and responsibly engage with the media they consume and produce (e.g., chatbots and social media influencers as sources of sexual health information; identifying and reporting AI-generated revenge porn; sexting; using dating apps). MLE scholars and practitioners must reflect on how new technologies will be used in the future - by marketers, media companies, and youth - and their repercussions on adolescent sexual health. Media can be important sources of sexual health information, powerful agents for sexual health promotion, and can provide safe spaces and community for marginalized groups, such as sexual and gender minority youth. In the age of digital misinformation and disinformation, MLE can teach adolescents the skills to effectively search for and evaluate the accuracy of sexual health information. Furthermore, adolescents are media producers. MLE must expand to equip students with the skills to safely create and disseminate media content, while fostering an understanding of the consequences – positive and negative – that can result from the media they produce and share. The constantly evolving media environment offers a dynamic space for researchers, educators, and youth to shape MLE programs that will empower adolescents to resist potentially harmful media influence, counter unhealthy mainstream messages about sex, effectively navigate media to enhance their sexual development and health, and become responsible media producers.

Note

1 Additional program evaluations have been conducted (see Maness et al., 2022; Scull et al., 2021; Scull et al., 2014), but are not the focus of this chapter.

References

Ajzen, I. (1991). The theory of planned behavior. *Organizational Behavior and Human Decision Processes*, *50*, 179–211. https://doi.org/10.1016/0749-5978(91)90020-T

Austin, E. W., & Johnson, K. K. (1997). Effects of general and alcohol–specific media literacy training on children's decision making about alcohol. *Journal of Health Communication*, *2*, 17–42. https://doi.org/10.1080/108107397127897

Baams, L., Overbeek, G., Dubas, J. S., Doornwaard, S. M., Rommes, E., & Van Aken, M. A. (2015). Perceived realism moderates the relation between sexualized media consumption and permissive sexual attitudes in Dutch adolescents. *Archives of Sexual Behavior*, *44*(3), 743–754.

Basen-Engquist, K., Masse, L. C., Coyle, K., Kirby, D., Parcel, G. S., Banspach, S., & Nodora, J. (1999). Validity of scales measuring the psychosocial determinants of HIV/STD-related risk behavior in adolescents. *Health Education Research*, *14*(1), 25–38.

Brown, J. D. (2006). Media literacy has potential to improve adolescents' health. *Journal of Adolescent Health*, *39*(4), 459–460. https://doi.org/10.1016/j.jadohealth.2006.07.014

Buhi, E. R., & Goodson, P. (2007). Predictors of adolescent sexual behavior and intention: a theory-guided systematic review. *Journal of Adolescent Health*, *40*(1), 4–21. https://doi.org/10.1016/j.jadohealth.2006.09.027

Busselle, R. W., & Greenberg, B. S. (2000). The nature of television realism judgments: A reevaluation of their conceptualization and measurement. *Mass Communication & Society*, *3*(2–3), 249–268. https://doi.org/10.1207/S15327825MCS0323_05

Chaiken, S., & Trope, Y. (1999). *Dual-process theories in social psychology*. Guilford Press.

Collier, K. M., Coyne, S. M., Rasmussen, E. E., Hawkins, A. J., Padilla-Walker, L. M., Erickson, S. E., & Memmott-Elison, M. K. (2016). Does parental mediation of media influence child outcomes? A meta-analysis on media time, aggression, substance use, and sexual behavior. *Developmental Psychology, 52*(5), 798–812. https://doi.org/10.1037/dev0000108

Coyne, S. M., Ward, L. M., Kroff, S. L., Davis, E. J., Holmgren, H. G., Jensen, A. C., Erickson, S. E., & Essig, L. W. (2019). Contributions of mainstream sexual media exposure to sexual attitudes, perceived peer norms, and sexual behavior: A meta-analysis. *Journal of Adolescent Health*. https://doi.org/10.1016/j.jadohealth.2018.11.016

Dillman Carpentier, F. R., Stevens, E. M., Wu, L., & Seely, N. (2017). Sex, love, and risk-n-responsibility: A content analysis of entertainment television. *Mass Communication and Society, 20*(5), 686–709. https://doi.org/10.1080/15205436.2017.1298807

Dodson, C. V., Scull, T. M., & Kupersmidt, J. B. (2024). Quantitative methods for assessing media literacy in evaluations of health promotion intervention programs using media literacy education. In P. Fastrez, N. Landry (ed.), *Media Literacy and Media Education Research Methods: A Handbook*. Routledge.

Evans-Paulson, R., Dodson, C. V., & Scull, T. M. (2023). Critical media attitudes as a buffer against the harmful effects of pornography on beliefs about sexual and dating violence. *Sex Education*, 1–17. https://doi.org/10.1080/14681811.2023.2241133

Foshee, V. A., Bauman, K. E., Ennett, S. T., Suchindran, C., Benefield, T., & Linder, G. F. (2005). Assessing the effects of the dating violence prevention program "Safe Dates" using random coefficient regression modeling. *Prevention Science, 6*(3), 245–258. https://doi.org/10.1007/s11121-005-0007-0

Gabarron, E., & Wynn, R. (2016). Use of social media for sexual health promotion: a scoping review. *Global Health Action, 9*, 32193. https://doi.org/10.3402/gha.v9.32193

Gibbons, F. X., Gerrard, M., Blanton, H., & Russell, D. W. (1998). Reasoned action and social reaction: Willingness and intention as independent predictors of health risk. *Journal of Personality and Social Psychology, 74*(5), 1164–1180. https://doi.org/10.1037/0022-3514.74.5.1164

Guttmacher Institute. (2023, September 1). *Sex and HIV Education: State Laws and Policies*. Retrieved April 4, 2024 from https://www.guttmacher.org/state-policy/explore/sex-and-hiv-education

Halpern-Felsher, B. L., Kropp, R. Y., Boyer, C. B., Tschann, J. M., & Ellen, J. M. (2004). Adolescents' self-efficacy to communicate about sex: Its role in condom attitudes, commitment, and use. *Adolescence, 39*(155), 443–456.

Hedrick, A. (2021). A meta-analysis of media consumption and rape myth acceptance. *Journal of Health Communication, 26*(9), 645–656. https://doi.org/10.1080/10810730.2021.1986609

Hobbs, R., & Jensen, A. (2009). The past present and future of media literacy education. *Journal of Media Literacy Education, 1*(11). https://doi.org/10.23860/jmle-1-1-1

Jeong, S. H., Cho, H., & Hwang, Y. (2012). Media literacy interventions: A meta-analytic review. *Journal of Communication*, 62(3), 454–472. https://doi.org/10.1111/j.1460-2466.2012.01643.x

Kupersmidt, J. B., Scull, T. M., & Austin, E. W. (2010). Media literacy education for elementary school substance use prevention: Study of Media Detective. *Pediatrics*, 126(3), 525–531. https://doi.org/10.1542/peds.2010-0068

Lou, C., & Kim, H. K. (2019). Fancying the new rich and famous? Explicating the roles of influencer content, credibility, and parental mediation in adolescents' parasocial relationship, materialism, and purchase intentions. *Frontiers in Psychology*, 10. https://doi.org/10.3389/fpsyg.2019.02567

Maness, S.B., Kershner, S.H., George, T.P., Pozsik, J.T., Gibson, M., & Marcano, D. (2022). Evaluation of a media literacy education program for sexual health promotion in older adolescents implemented in Southern universities. *Journal of American College Health*, 1–7. https://doi.org/10.1080/07448481.2022.2083917

McMahon, S., & Farmer, L. (2011). An updated measure for assessing subtle rape myths. *National Association of Social Workers*, 35(2), 71–81. http://www.jstor.org/stable/42659785

Myklestad, I., & Rise, J. (2007). Predicting willingness to engage in unsafe sex and intention to perform sexual protective behaviors among adolescents. *Health Education & Behavior*, 34(4), 686–699. https://doi.org/10.1177/1090198106289571

National Association for Media Literacy Education. (2024). *What is media literacy?* https://namle.org/resources/media-literacy-defined/

Peter, J., & Valkenburg, P. M. (2016). Adolescents' exposure to sexually explicit material on the internet. *Communication Research*, 33(2), 178–204. https://doi.org/10.1177/0093650205285369

Petty, R. E., & Cacioppo, J. T. (1986). The elaboration likelihood model of persuasion. In Springer Series in Social Psychology (ed.), *Communication and Persuasion*. Springer.

Reyes, H. L. M., Foshee, V. A., Niolon, P. H., Reidy, D. E., & Hall, J. E. (2016). Gender role attitudes and male adolescent dating violence perpetration: Normative beliefs as moderators. *Journal of Youth and Adolescence*, 45(2), 350–360. https://doi.org/10.1007/s10964-015-0278-0

Schouten, A. P., Janssen, L., & Verspaget, M. (2021). Celebrity vs. influencer endorsements in advertising: The role of identification, credibility, and product-endorser fit. In S. Yoon, Y. K. Choi, & C. R. Taylor (Eds.), *Leveraged Marketing Communications*. Routledge.

Scull, T. M., Dodson, C. V., Geller, J. G., Reeder, L., & Stump, K. N. (2022). A media literacy education approach to high school sexual health education: Effects of Media Aware on adolescents' media, sexual health, and communication outcomes. *Journal of Youth and Adolescence*, 51(4), 708–723. https://doi.org/10.1007/s10964-021-01567-0

Scull, T. M., Kupersmidt, J. B., Malik, C. V., & Keefe, E. M. (2018). Examining the efficacy of an mHealth media literacy education program for sexual health promotion in older adolescents attending community college. *Journal of American College Health*, 66(3), 165–177. https://doi.org/10.1080/07448481.2017.1393822

Scull, T. M., Kupersmidt, J. B., Malik, C. V., & Morgan-Lopez, A. A. (2018). Using media literacy education for adolescent sexual health promotion in middle school: Randomized control trial of Media Aware. *Journal of Health Communication*, 23(12), 1051–1063. https://doi.org/10.1080/10810730.2018.1548669

Scull, T. M., & Malik, C. V. (2019). Role of entertainment media in sexual socialization. In *The International Encyclopedia of Media Literacy* (pp. 1–11). https://doi.org/10.1002/9781118978238.ieml0214

Scull, T. M., Malik, C. V., & Kupersmidt, J. B. (2014). A media literacy education approach to teaching adolescents comprehensive sexual health education. *Journal of Media Literacy Education*, 6(1), 1–14.

Scull, T. M., Malik, C. V., & Kupersmidt, J. B. (2018). Understanding the unique role of media message processing in predicting adolescent sexual behavior intentions in the United States. *Journal of Children and Media*, 12(3), 258–274. https://doi.org/10.1080/17482798.2017.1403937

Scull, T. T. M., Malik, C. V., Morrison, A., & Keefe, E. (2021). Promoting sexual health in high school: A feasibility study of a web-based media literacy education program. *Journal of Health Communication*, 26(3), 147–160. https://doi.org/10.1080/10810730.2021.1893868

Sheeran, P., Maki, A., Montanaro, E., Avishai-Yitshak, A., Bryan, A., Klein, W. M. P., Miles, E., & Rothman, A. J. (2016). The impact of changing attitudes, norms, and self-efficacy on health-related intentions and behavior: A meta-analysis. *Health Psychology*, 35(11), 1178–1188. https://doi.org/10.1037/hea0000387

SIECUS. (2024). *State profiles*. Retrieved March 1, 2024, from https://siecus.org/state-profiles/

Tsfati, Y. (2003). Media skepticism and climate of opinion perception. *International Journal of Public Opinion Research*, 15(1), 65–82. https://doi.org/10.1093/ijpor/15.1.65

Turchik, J. A., & Garske, J. P. (2008). Measurement of sexual risk taking among college students. *Archives of Sexual Behavior*, 38(6), 936–948.

United States Food and Drug Administration. (2023). *Birth Control*. Retrieved March 1, 2024, from www.fda.gov/consumers/free-publications-women/birth-control#LARC

Vahedi, Z., Sibalis, A., & Sutherland, J. E. (2018). Are media literacy interventions effective at changing attitudes and intentions towards risky health behaviors in adolescents? A meta-analytic review. *Journal of Adolescence*, 67, 140–152. https://doi.org/10.1016/j.adolescence.2018.06.007

Ward, L. M. (2003). Understanding the role of entertainment media in the sexual socialization of American youth: A review of empirical research. *Developmental Review*, 23(3), 347–388. https://doi.org/10.1016/s0273-2297(03)00013-3

Ward, L. M., Erickson, S. E., Lippman, J., & Giaccardi, S. (2016). Sexual media content and effects. In J. F. Nussbaum (ed.), *Oxford Research Encyclopedia of Communication* (Vol. 1): Oxford University Press.

Ward, L. M., & Grower, P. (2020). Media and the development of gender role stereotypes. *Annual Review of Developmental Psychology*, 2, 177–199. https://doi.org/10.1146/annurev-devpsych-051120-010630

Ward, L. M., Moorman, J. D., & Grower, P. (2019). Entertainment media's role in the sexual socialization of Western youth: A review of research from

2000–2017. In S. L. J. Gilbert (ed.), *The Cambridge handbook of sexual development: Childhood and adolescence* (pp. 395–418). Cambridge University Press.

Wright, P. J. (2009). Sexual socialization messages in mainstream entertainment mass media: A review and synthesis. *Sexuality & Culture, 13*(4), 181–200. https://doi.org/10.1007/s12119-009-9050-5

Wright, P. J., Herbenick, D., & Paul, B. (2022). Casual condomless sex, range of pornography exposure, and perceived pornography realism. *Communication Research, 49*(4), 547–566. https://doi.org/10.1177/00936502211003765

Xie, X., Gai, X., & Zhou, Y. (2019). A meta-analysis of media literacy interventions for deviant behaviors. *Computers & Education, 139,* 146–156. https://doi.org/10.1016/j.compedu.2019.05.008

Yapp, E. J., & Quayle, E. (2018). A systematic review of the association between rape myth acceptance and male-on-female sexual violence. *Aggression and Violent Behavior, 41,* 1–19. https://doi.org/10.1016/j.avb.2018.05.002

17

PARTICIPATORY PATHWAYS

Envisioning Youth-Centric Digital Sexual Health Education

Carina M. Zelaya, Rachell Hanebutt, and Angela Cooke-Jackson

In today's digital era, sexuality and sexual health information increasingly migrate online posing both opportunities and hurdles, especially for youth seeking knowledge on digital platforms. Multiple studies that document this trend underscore the changing dynamics of accessing and disseminating sexual health information (Holstrom, 2015; Manduley et al., 2018; Nikkelen et al., 2019). Adolescents and young adults now have access to diverse sources, from official government websites to social media and online influencers. This digital shift in sexual health education offers privacy and anonymity, with information shared across various platforms like websites, text messages, digital stories, and mobile apps.

In response to this shift, in 2011, major organizations, including the Internet Sexuality Information Services (ISIS), National Institute of Mental Health (NIMH), and the Ford Foundation, brought together more than 50 scientists and technology specialists to explore new, innovative technological approaches for sexuality and sexual health education in the United States. As Allison et al. (2012) noted in their report, the meeting highlighted a significant gap in research on the development and evaluation of digital strategies for safer sexual health practices among young people. Despite these efforts, more than a decade later, challenges remain in assessing the quality and relevance of these digital resources for younger audiences in the United States (Diez et al., 2022). For instance, recent studies suggest that current digital materials may not adequately prepare young people for a healthy sexual life (Andrzejewski et al., 2020; Sewak et al., 2023).

Building on this premise, the current study was conducted to understand what information young adults wished they had about sexuality and

DOI: 10.4324/9781032648880-21

sexual health online when they were younger. Informed by Bailey et al.'s (2015) recommendation, our study promotes young adults' active participation in developing educational content, drawing from their past experiences and specific information needs. This approach aims to tailor digital resources more precisely to the diverse needs of youth to ensure that these platforms are not just informative but also empowering.

The digital transformation of sexual health promotion

The shift of young adults toward digital media for sexuality and sexual health information is, in many ways, a response to the inadequacies of school-based sex education systems present in the United States (Cooke-Jackson et al., 2021). Studies show that these strategies are often outdated and do not fully address the complex sexual realities of young people (Astle et al., 2021; Charest et al., 2016). Consequently, young adults increasingly turn to online sources in search of more relevant, up-to-date, and comprehensive information (Astle et al., 2021; Baker et al., 2021; Plaisime et al., 2020). This disconnect between formal education and young people's realities places a growing responsibility on online sexuality and sexual health resources as they have evolved from supplementary sources to becoming primary conduits for delivering sexuality and sexual health content (Nikkelen et al., 2019; Bailey et al., 2015).

Young people are also drawn to digital platforms because they provide quick and easy access to information (Engel, 2023; Flanders et al., 2021). However, the ease of accessing these platforms often brings challenges, especially in verifying the accuracy and appropriateness of content (Andrzejewski et al., 2020; Rothman et al., 2021). Notably, prior research has documented a gap in the availability of reliable, age-appropriate advice on relationship management and sexual decision-making within online resources (Patterson et al., 2019; Plaisime et al., 2020). For instance, in their study, Patterson et al. (2019) discovered that young people experienced challenges such as exposure to an overabundance of content, concerns about the trustworthiness of sources, struggles in locating local services, and apprehensions about privacy and engaging with visual or auditory materials, all of which deterred them from accessing sexual health information online. Therefore, additional research is needed to pinpoint strategies that could enhance digital platforms dedicated to enriching sexuality and sexual health education.

Meeting sexual and gender diversity needs

Despite advances in promoting diversity, equity, and inclusion (DEI) in sexuality and sexual health education in the United States, a significant gap in research persists regarding the effectiveness of available online resources in meeting the needs of sexual and gender minority (SGM) youth[1]. Although content related to sexual and gender diversity is available across digital platforms, it often lacks depth and fails to meet the complex needs of diverse youth populations, rarely going beyond basic definitions to explore the complex realities faced by individuals who do not conform to mainstream sexual norms (Andrzejewski et al., 2020; Hanebutt, 2021). Studies have also critiqued the accessibility and applicability of the information available online. A scoping review by Baker et al. (2021), for example, examined a broad range of digital media interventions aimed at promoting sexual health among young people and found that many digital resources do not adequately address the needs of sexually and gender-diverse populations. Their research suggests that while digital platforms have the potential to reach a wide audience, they frequently miss the opportunity to provide inclusive and comprehensive education.

Method

We recruited 300 participants, aged 18–24 (M = 22.36, SD = 1.68), from the United States via the survey sampling company Prolific. We surveyed 142 (47.3%) females, 129 (43%) males, and 29 (9.7%) non-binary people. Participants were allowed to select multiple racial identities, resulting in the following breakdown: 180 (61%) selected White, 54 (18%) selected Asian/Asian-American/Pacific Islander, 43 (14%) selected Black/African American, 40 (13%) selected Hispanic/Latine, and 2 (1%) selected Native American or Alaska Native. In terms of sexual orientation, 153 (51.5%) identified as heterosexual, 71 (24%) identified as bi-sexual, 49 (16.5%) identified as gay/lesbian, 13 (4%) identified as pansexual, 7 (2%) identified as asexual, and 7 (2%) chose not to disclose.

Our study analyzed a specific set of data derived from a broader cross-sectional survey in the United States. Drawing inspiration from recent research (Astle et al., 2021; Baker et al., 2021; Kuborn et al., 2023; Rubinsky & Cooke-Jackson, 2017), we asked participants, in an open-ended format, to think back to their younger years and identify the sexuality and sexual health information they wish they had accessed online during that time. Before participating, each participant gave their informed consent. After completing the survey, they were asked to fill out a short demographic questionnaire. Participants received compensation via the Prolific platform. The study was approved by the first author's Institutional Review Board. This study received funding from the University of Maryland's College of Arts and Humanities Faculty Fund Award.

We began by using descriptive statistics to summarize the participants' demographic data. For the qualitative component, we conducted a thematic analysis following the framework outlined by Braun and Clarke (2012). According to Braun and Clarke, thematic analysis "is a method for systematically identifying, organizing, and offering insight into patterns of meaning (themes) across a dataset" (p. 57). It serves as a method for identifying commonalities in the discussion or written expression of topics and for understanding the significance of those commonalities. We used an inductive approach, which allowed us to explore the participants' insights flexibly and uncover themes that were not initially expected (Saldaña, 2021). The responses from the participants typically ranged from 50- to 300-word responses. The lead author identified key themes and systematically coded the responses. Throughout the analysis and interpretation stages, the research team engaged in discussions, offered feedback, and reached a consensus on the findings.

Results

Three major themes emerged from the analysis, each representing a distinct aspect of sexual health information that participants wished had been more accessible during their teenage years: a) actionable guidance on sexual activities, b) authentic depictions of sexual anatomy, and c) diverse and inclusive sexual discourse. The demographic information provided in the quotes reflects the self-reported identities of the participants.

Actionable guidance on sexual activities

The predominant theme from the participants revolved around the need for practical and detailed guidance on sexual activities. Moreover, participants pointed out a deficiency in online resources where fundamental aspects of engaging in sexual experiences are overlooked, inaccurately portrayed, or obscured by ambiguity. For example, a 22-year-old White, straight, cisgender man lamented the lack of "official websites that talked about sex in a detailed manner or had pictures showcasing the specifics." Participants also voiced a need for guidance that sets realistic expectations about sexual experiences, particularly for those engaging in sex for the first time. A 22-year-old Black, straight, cisgender woman shared:

> I wish I had found more information about what sex was like, what to expect when first having sex and the guilt of losing or not losing one's virginity. Feeling ready for sex and how to know when is the "right" time.

The challenge of navigating sexual education online was further compounded by the nature of available content. A 21-year-old Asian, nonbinary participant pointed out their failed quest for authentic and relatable content:

> Official sites usually don't talk about people's own personal sexual experiences in a direct and detailed manner, they always just highlight the risks of having sex or happy endings, it felt generic and didn't feel real so it was hard to take an example from.

Similarly, a 24-year-old Black, gay, cisgender man shared:

> There's a lot of the stuff that isn't as serious or health related like having sex is either a meme/joke or sexually explicit content that isn't necessarily intended to educate. This can make it difficult to learn purely about sex.

These sentiments were echoed by others, with many feeling that the available resources failed to connect on a personal or practical level.

Importantly, participants expressed a need for better resources on female sexual pleasure and females achieving orgasm. For instance, a 21-year-old White, straight, cisgender woman shared her personal struggle:

> I felt super insecure and felt like I was a part of the small percentage of women who were not able to orgasm. This information would have helped me feel better by allowing me to learn how to explore my body better, how to feel comfortable doing so, and not making me feel guilty when my partner is trying to help.

Similarly, a 24-year-old Black-Latino, straight, cisgender man longed for information on "how to make sex pleasurable for a woman and meeting their needs when it comes to sex," adding that such knowledge "would have saved me some awkward interactions with women and would have made me more in tune with women."

Authentic depictions of sexual anatomy

Another prominent theme we identified among our participants was the difficulty in accessing clear and body-positive information about sexual anatomy that is easy to understand and acknowledge the diversity of human bodies. For example, a 23-year-old, White, straight, cisgender woman noted, "I would have liked to know more about anatomical information... it would have been useful to deal with puberty and self-discovery." This desire for clearer, more detailed explanations was stated by others as well, including a 20-year-old White, gay, cisgender man who shared, "I wished I had come across more information about very basic differences in penis anatomy, I mean, it was only until I was around 16 that I even learned I didn't have a natural penis."

Many participants voiced concerns over not understanding the normal appearance of genitalia. A 20-year-old Black, lesbian, cisgender woman shared, "I didn't understand what a vagina was supposed to look like and if the color and shape of mine were normal." The limited or biased portrayal of sexual anatomy was also said to affect participants' body image and self-esteem. A 19-year-old White, straight, cisgender woman wished there had been more information available about "the diversity of female bodies in my teenage years and the variations in normal anatomy, as I felt insecure about things like my breasts and labia." Similarly, a 22-year-old Asian, gay, cisgender man noted, "Having any relevant body positive information on penis size would have helped me to avoid obsessing over it."

Diverse and inclusive sexual discourse

Participants commonly expressed concerns about the digital sexual health resources being predominantly influenced by heteronormative and male-centric views, often overlooking female pleasure and the varied experiences of sexual and gender minorities. For example, a 20-year-old White, bi-sexual, cisgender woman highlighted the challenge of "finding information provided from a woman-centric perspective, especially considering a lot of patriarchal ideas can slip into the ways non-men view sexual health." This issue of representation and relevance was also noted by a 23-year-old, Black, bi-sexual cisgender woman who found content "too broad, and not as relevant to me as a cisgender woman in a non-monogamous queer relationship." A 19-year-old White, lesbian, cisgender woman also shared, "queer experiences are stigmatized and thought to be 'funny.' Often, it furthers a certain heterosexual dynamic."

The lack of content accurately reflecting the lives of queer, trans, and non-binary individuals was a significant concern. An 18-year-old Black trans participant yearned for "any information on how trans people had sex and experienced pleasure in a way that was not through pornography." They reflected, "I would have been able to better understand myself and others in sexual relationships." Participants unequivocally shared this desire for reliable, accessible information. For instance, one 23-year-old White, gay, cisgender man sought "frank and honest information from a trusted source about gay sex." Questions around the concept of virginity in queer relationships were also raised, with a 20-year-old White, lesbian, cisgender woman seeking clarity on "the construct of virginity and queer sex," while a 19-year-old White, lesbian, cisgender woman inquired about the necessity of dental dams for "two virgin lesbians."

A significant number of participants voiced a need for greater awareness and understanding of asexuality. One 24-year-old White, asexual, cisgender woman wished for earlier exposure to the concept of asexuality to "have understood myself better, and what this might mean for my own sexual health." The desire for more comprehensive and inclusive information regarding asexuality was reiterated by a 22-year-old Black, asexual, cisgender man who emphasized, "I knew people in online spaces at the time who were asexual but there wasn't as much information when I was younger about what that means and the spectrum of experiences that covers." Lastly, one 20-year-old White, asexual, non-binary individual poignantly shared:

At the time, there wasn't much information on asexuality online. It is much better now, though. But if it had been accessible sooner, I wouldn't have spent 5 years forcing myself to try and enjoy sex when I never have and never will.

Discussion

The digital revolution has significantly transformed sexual health education in the United States. Although digital platforms offer unprecedented access to information, our study underscores the persistent shortcomings in addressing the varied needs of individuals seeking sexual health information online, particularly among adolescents. This challenge is not unique to U.S. adolescents, as teens globally face similar obstacles in accessing reliable sexual health information, suggesting a universal need to overhaul how sexual education is delivered (Bailey et al., 2015; Patterson et al., 2019).

Embrace a holistic educational approach

A key finding in our study is the demand for sexual health education that moves beyond the traditional, risk-averse narratives. Participants called for a more holistic approach that incorporates discussions of pleasure, emotional intimacy, and the social contexts of sexual experiences, resonating with findings from Kuborn et al. (2023) and Astle et al. (2021). This aligns with recent scholarship advocating for a broader, more positive approach to sex education that includes pleasure and desire as core components (Rubinsky & Cooke-Jackson, 2017; Harvey et al., 2023). Educators, policymakers, and digital content creators are urged to transition from traditional narratives centered on risks to a broader perspective that acknowledges pleasure, desire, and the emotional and social dimensions of sexual experiences. By embracing this approach, powerholders can equip individuals with actionable advice, help set realistic expectations, and celebrate the diversity of sexual experiences.

Showcase authentic sexual experiences and anatomy

In addressing the pressing need for comprehensive sexual health education, it's crucial to ensure that educational materials provide inclusive, body-positive information about sexual anatomy, particularly concerning genitalia. Mainstream media and pornography often perpetuate narrow and biased depictions of sexual organs, exacerbating this challenge (Baker et al., 2021; Harvey et al., 2023; Waling et al., 2023). This observation resonates with prior research (Astle et al., 2021; Baker et al., 2021), which underscores the importance of accurate, body-positive information in combating societal norms and nurturing positive self-esteem and body image. To tackle these shortcomings, powerholders must focus on crafting content that authentically portrays sexual experiences and offers inclusive, body-positive information about sexual anatomy. By doing so, they can challenge the myths propagated by explicit media and celebrate the rich diversity of human bodies, thereby promoting positive body image and sexual fulfillment. Recognizing the positive impact of understanding natural genital diversity underscores the urgent need to integrate such content into sexual health resources. By aligning body-positive online content with a participatory health education approach (Baker et al., 2021), powerholders can cultivate a more holistic and accepting view of bodies in all their diversity, thereby fostering healthier attitudes and behaviors regarding sexual health.

Ensure inclusion for sexual and gender minorities

Participants from these communities expressed valid concerns regarding the lack of relevant and affirming information that speaks to their unique experiences and identities. This finding echoes broader issues within sexual health education, where queer, trans, non-binary, and asexual individuals often feel marginalized or overlooked. This also mirrors concerns raised by previous research highlighting the disparities in sexual health education for SGM individuals (Andrzejewski et al., 2020; Charest et al., 2016).

To address this gap, powerholders must take proactive steps to tailor sexual health resources to reflect the diverse experiences and identities of all users. This involves providing accurate information that acknowledges and affirms diverse identities, while also addressing the specific needs and challenges faced by sexual and gender minorities. By doing so, powerholders can create a more inclusive and supportive environment where all individuals can access vital sexual health information without fear of exclusion or discrimination. Initiatives like Queer Sex Ed (Mustanski et al., 2015) demonstrate how tailored digital resources can effectively bridge these gaps, improving knowledge and reducing disparities among SGM individuals. By leveraging such approaches and embracing the diversity of human experiences and identities, powerholders can work toward creating a more equitable and inclusive sexual health education landscape for all.

Collaborative content creation

Our study emphasizes the importance of cultivating collaboration and community involvement in the development of sexual health materials. By collaborating with communities, healthcare experts, educators, and content creators, powerholders can co-develop sexual health materials that are informed by the latest research, best practices, and the diverse experiences of various populations (Hanebutt, 2021). By working together, powerholders can ensure that the content is not only educational and trustworthy but also resonates with its intended audiences on a deeper level. In essence, collaborative content creation serves as a cornerstone for developing sexual health materials that are both informative and engaging, ultimately leading to better outcomes for individuals seeking sexual health information. By leveraging the collective wisdom and insights of various powerholders, we can create a more inclusive and impactful sexual health education landscape for all.

Our findings offer practical applications for educators, policymakers, and digital content creators, providing a roadmap for improving sexual health education in the digital realm. However, our study is not without limitations. The methodology and potential biases warrant careful consideration. The retrospective nature of participant reflections might be influenced by current perceptions and experiences, potentially coloring their accounts of past informational desires and gaps. Future research should aim to broaden the diversity of participants and digital spaces examined to ensure more comprehensive insights into digital sexual health education.

Our study underscores the significant role digital platforms play in reshaping sexual health education, calling for a strategic move toward content that is more inclusive, comprehensive, and user-centric.

In conclusion, the findings from our study underscore the pressing need for a strategic change of sexual health education content on digital platforms. The current landscape is characterized by a lack of inclusivity, comprehensiveness, and user-centricity, which hinders its effectiveness in addressing the diverse needs of individuals seeking sexual health information online. Therefore, we advocate for a deliberate shift toward developing content that is more inclusive, comprehensive, and tailored to the needs of users. To achieve this goal, powerholders must first recognize the importance of inclusivity. By acknowledging and affirming the experiences of sexual and gender minorities, as well as individuals from various cultural, ethnic, and socioeconomic backgrounds, content creators can create a more welcoming and supportive digital environment for all users. Additionally, the content should be user-centric, meaning that it is designed with the needs, preferences, and digital literacy levels of the target audience in mind. This requires engaging users in the content creation process, soliciting feedback, and adapting the content based on user input. Through collaborative efforts and a commitment to continuous improvement, we can create a digital sexual health education landscape that meets the diverse needs of users and contributes to positive sexual health outcomes for all.

Note

1 Note on terminology: Although "SGM" and "LGBTQ+" are often used interchangeably, this chapter will use "SGM" as it more inclusively represents a broader spectrum of evolving sexual and gender identities.

References

Allison, S., Bauermeister, J. A., Bull, S., Lightfoot, M., Mustanski, B., Shegog, R., & Levine, D. (2012). The intersection of youth, technology, and new media with sexual health: Moving the research agenda forward. *Journal of Adolescent Health*, 51(3), 207–212. https://doi.org/10.1016/j.jadohealth.2012.06.012

Andrzejewski, J., Rasberry, C. N., Mustanski, B., & Steiner, R. J. (2020). Sexual and reproductive health websites: An analysis of content for sexual and gender minority youth. *American Journal of Health Promotion*, 34(4), 393–401. https://doi.org/10.1177/0890117119899217

Astle, S., McAllister, P., Emanuels, S., Rogers, J., Toews, M., & Yazedjian, A. (2021). College students' suggestions for improving sex education in schools beyond 'blah blah blah condoms and STDs'. *Sex Education*, 21(1), 91–105. https://doi.org/10.1080/14681811.2020.1749044

Bailey, J., Mann, S., Wayal, S., Hunter, R., Free, C., Abraham, C., & Murray, E. (2015). Sexual health promotion for young people delivered via digital media: A scoping review. *Public Health Research*, 3(13), 1–119. https://doi.org/10.3310/phr03130

Baker, A. M., Jahn, J. L., Tan, A. S., Katz-Wise, S. L., Viswanath, K., Bishop, R. A., & Agénor, M. (2021). Sexual health information sources, needs, and preferences of young adult sexual minority cisgender women and non-binary individuals assigned female at birth. *Sexuality Research and Social Policy, 18*, 775–787. https://doi.org/10.1007/s13178-020-00501-6

Braun, V. & Clarke, V. (2012) Thematic analysis. In H. Cooper, P. M. Camic, D. L. Long, A. T. Panter, D. Rindskopf, & K. J. Sher (eds.), *APA Handbook of Research Methods in Psychology, Vol. 2: Research designs: Quantitative, qualitative, neuropsychological, and biological* (pp. 57–71). Washington, D.C: American Psychological Association.

Charest, M., Kleinplatz, P. J., & Lund, J. I. (2016). Sexual health information disparities between heterosexual and LGBTQ+ young adults: Implications for sexual health. *The Canadian Journal of Human Sexuality, 25*(2), 74–85. https://doi.org/10.3138/cjhs.252-A9

Cooke-Jackson, A., McMahon, T., & Shah, K. (2021). Intimate communication guidelines for transformative sexual education. In A. Cooke-Jackson & V. Rubinsky (eds.), *Communicating Intimate Health* (pp. 63–72). Rowman & Littlefield.

Diez, S. L., Fava, N. M., Fernandez, S. B., & Mendel, W. E. (2022). Sexual health education: The untapped and unmeasured potential of US-based websites. *Sex Education, 22*(3), 335–347. https://doi.org/10.1080/14681811.2021.1935227

Engel, E. (2023). Young peoples' perceived benefits and barriers of sexual health promotion on social media - a literature review. *International Journal of Health Promotion and Education*, 1–20. https://doi.org/10.1080/14635240.2023.2241035

Flanders, C. E., Dinh, R. N., Pragg, L., Dobinson, C., & Logie, C. H. (2021). Young sexual minority women's evaluation processes of online and digital sexual health information. *Health Communication, 36*(10), 1286–1294. https://doi.org/10.1080/10410236.2020.1751381

Hanebutt, R. (2021). Beyond the binaries of sexual consent. In A. Cooke-Jackson & V. Rubinsky (eds.), *Communicating Intimate Health* (pp. 99–118). Lexington Books. https://rowman.com/ISBN/ 9781793630971/ Communicating-Intimate-Health

Harvey, P., Jones, E., & Copulsky, D. (2023). The relational nature of gender, the pervasiveness of heteronormative sexual scripts, and the impact on sexual pleasure. *Archives of Sexual Behavior, 52*(3), 1195–1212. https://doi.org/10.1007/s10508-023-02558-x

Holstrom, A. M. (2015). Sexuality education goes viral: What we know about online sexual health information. *American Journal of Sexuality Education, 10*(3), 277–294. http://dx.doi.org/10.1080/15546128.2015.1040569

Kuborn, S., Markham, M., & Astle, S. (2023). "I wish I had been told the truth sooner": The sexuality education college women wish they had. *Sexuality Research and Social Policy*, 1–15. https://doi.org/10.1007/s13178-023-00887-z

Manduley, A. E., Mertens, A., Plante, I., & Sultana, A. (2018). The role of social media in sex education: Dispatches from queer, trans, and racialized communities. *Feminism & Psychology, 28*(1), 152–170. https://doi.org/10.1177/0959353517717751

Mustanski, B., Greene, G. J., Ryan, D., & Whitton, S. W. (2015). Feasibility, acceptability, and initial efficacy of an online sexual health promotion program for LGBT youth: The Queer Sex Ed intervention. *The Journal of Sex Research*, 52(2), 220–230. https://doi.org/10.1080/00224499.2013.867924

Nikkelen, S. W., van Oosten, J. M., & van den Borne, M. M. (2019). Sexuality education in the digital era: Intrinsic and extrinsic predictors of online sexual information seeking among youth. *The Journal of Sex Research*, 57(2), 189–199. https://doi.org/10.1080/00224499.2019.1612830

Patterson, S. P., Hilton, S., Flowers, P., & McDaid, L. M. (2019). What are the barriers and challenges faced by adolescents when searching for sexual health information on the internet? Implications for policy and practice from a qualitative study. *Sexually Transmitted Infections*, 95, 462–467 https://doi.org/10.1136/sextrans-2018-053710

Plaisime, M., Robertson-James, C., Mejia, L., Núñez, A., Wolf, J., & Reels, S. (2020). Social media and teens: A needs assessment exploring the potential role of social media in promoting health. *Social Media + Society*, 6(1), 1–11. https://doi.org/10.1177/2056305119886025

Rothman, E. F., Beckmeyer, J. J., Herbenick, D., Fu, T. C., Dodge, B., & Fortenberry, J. D. (2021). The prevalence of using pornography for information about how to have sex: Findings from a nationally representative survey of US adolescents and young adults. *Archives of Sexual Behavior*, 50, 629–646. https://doi.org/10.1007/s10508-020-01877-7

Rubinsky, V., & Cooke-Jackson, A. (2017). "Tell me something other than to use a condom and sex is scary": Memorable messages women and gender minorities wish for and recall about sexual health. *Women's Studies in Communication*, 40(4), 379–400. https://doi.org/10.1080/07491409.2017.1368761

Saldaña, J. (2021). *The coding manual for qualitative researchers*. Sage Publications.

Sewak, A., Yousef, M., Deshpande, S., Seydel, T., & Hashemi, N. (2023). The effectiveness of digital sexual health interventions for young adults: A systematic literature review (2010–2020). *Health Promotion International*, 38(1), 1–14. https://doi.org/10.1093/heapro/daac104

Waling, A., Farrugia, A., & Fraser, S. (2023). Embarrassment, shame, and reassurance: Emotion and young people's access to online sexual health information. *Sexuality Research and Social Policy*, 20, 45–57. https://doi.org/10.1007/s13178-021-00668-6

18

DISCLOSURE OF SEXUAL ASSAULT IN ENTERTAINMENT MEDIA

Adolescent Girls' Sense-Making of Supportive and Unsupportive Sexual Assault Disclosure Narratives

Rachel E. Riggs, Sydney E. Brammer, and Rochelle R. Davidson Mhonde

Sexual assault victimization (SAV) increases in prevalence during adolescence for girls, and by the time they reach 17 years of age, more than one out of nine girls in the United States have experienced sexual abuse or sexual assault (Finkelhor et al., 2014). SAV disclosure motivations and help-seeking behaviors are under-researched in adolescent populations (Campbell et al., 2015), even though disclosure of SAV to a trusted adult or parent is key for adolescent girls to access social support and medical care (Kaufman, 2008). Critically, adolescent girls face unique barriers to disclosing as compared to other age groups (i.e., adult women), such as fear of repercussions for "bringing trouble onto the family" (McElvaney et al., 2014, p. 930) due to a false sense of complicity in the abuse and its consequences (Goodman-Brown et al., 2003). This chapter focused specifically on how adolescent girls in the United States made sense of SAV disclosure narratives in entertainment media, as girls under the age of 18 experience sexual assault at alarming rates (Finkelhor et al., 2014).

Many adolescents turn to media for information about sexual health topics, such as sexual assault, and media with sexual content can influence teenagers' and young adults' attitudes and thoughts about sex (Coyne et al., 2019). Exposure to SAV narratives in media may therefore help adolescents make sense of these experiences and how they might respond in the future, using narrative sense-making, especially if they have similar past experiences (Koenig Kellas, 2017). This chapter, therefore, investigates how adolescent girls understand and relate to SAV narratives in the media, specifically when exposed to assault disclosures where the victim/survivor is either

DOI: 10.4324/9781032648880-22

met with support from others (i.e., supportive disclosure), or receive blame and lack of support from others (i.e., unsupportive disclosure).

Television and sexual assault victimization narratives

Many adolescents in the United States have access to a vast media landscape, which boasts content of every genre and purpose imaginable, both in classic forms (e.g., movies, television) and nascent, digital formats (e.g., social media). Although it is a common assumption that young people have abandoned traditional media, 49% of U.S. adolescents report daily television viewership, and many have the television on in the background while engaging in other media activities (Rideout et al., 2022). A majority of 13- to 18-year-olds reported daily television viewership (55%) during the COVID-19 pandemic (Rideout et al., 2022), and many continue to report frequent engagement with outlets such as Netflix and YouTube post-pandemic (Sandler, 2022).

Popular television shows such as *13 Reasons Why* and *Sex Education* include numerous SAV narratives (i.e., storylines where characters either experience or discuss nonconsensual sexual experiences) and are marketed toward adolescent girls despite having TV-MA ratings (Seeberger et al., 2023). Serisier (2018) explains that SAV narratives—delivered in and through nearly every media format imaginable—place survivors in a unique position to potentially find disclosure empowering despite the vulnerability and risks that may simultaneously arise. Thus, further research into SAV narratives and how viewers make sense of those narratives (i.e., narrative sense-making) is critical, necessitated by the potential for media encounters to provide audiences with new perspectives and opportunities to learn and empathize (Murphy, 2021).

Adolescent sense-making about sexual assault

According to Koenig Kellas (2017), communicated narrative sense-making (CNSM) scholarship helps us understand the function of storytelling as connected to audience members' health in ways that may drive connection, learning, and coping. At its core, CNSM holds that rich narratives can effectively address difficult topics, including those that result in lasting trauma (Koenig Kellas, 2017; Koenig Kellas et al., 2020). This study uses the heuristic of retrospective storytelling of CNSM, focusing on the story's content, including how individuals perceive and share the content and the effect these perceptions have on beliefs, values, behaviors, and well-being (Koenig Kellas, 2017). Although most of the scholarship on CNSM examines storytelling and sharing in interpersonal relationships (Holman &

Koenig Kellas, 2018; Flood-Grady & Koenig Kellas, 2019), we used televised stories as retrospective content for this study to provide insight into how media tells the story of sexual assault. Furthermore, CNSM offers a framework for analysis of the values and cultural scripts related to sexual assault that are interpreted in the viewing of media.

When individuals engage in the narrative process to understand a health issue (i.e., construct a story about their health experiences), they can connect related facts and make sense of information more effectively (Pennebaker, 2000). Adolescents and young adults are tasked with making sense of their childhood experiences as they prepare for adulthood (McAdams, 2001), so narrative sense-making is often key for positive well-being among young adults (Schwartz et al., 2005). For adolescents, it is important to understand how they make sense of traumatic situations like SAV because negative health outcomes (e.g., depression and post-traumatic stress disorder) following traumatic experiences can last well into adulthood (Dunn et al., 2016). For example, Horstman (2019) found that young adult women often write about recognizing struggles, taking steps to solve problems, looking for the positives, and finding strength in relationships when making sense of difficult situations.

Adolescent girls' self-efficacy and disclosure narratives

Bandura (2001) describes self-efficacy as the degree to which one believes that they can accomplish an action they plan to attempt. Self-efficacy is not fixed; it can change over time and is often developed in adolescence (Pajares, 2005). Adolescents may "have little incentive to act or to persevere in the face of the difficulties that inevitably ensue" (p. 339) unless they have self-efficacy and believe that their actions will produce the desired outcomes (Pajares, 2005). Importantly, one potential marker of positive sense-making is one's ability to tell her story despite hardships. Thus, adolescent girls' self-efficacy beliefs could influence their ability to disclose SAV. For example, previous research has found that mediated SAV narratives featuring self-efficacy messages may encourage adolescents to feel more self-efficacious in disclosing their assaults (Riggs & Rasmussen, 2021).

Adolescent victims often consider the responses of their peers and families when they consider disclosing information about sexual assault (Ullman, 2024). Others' responses to disclosures also matters to victims when they consider disclosing information about their sexual assault in the future (Ahrens et al., 2010). Negative, unsupportive responses, like controlling the victim's autonomy or blaming the victim, can lead to negative outcomes for the victim (Orchowski et al., 2013). Campbell et al. (2015) found that victims who received positive support (i.e., reassurance, coping, and believing) were more likely to have positive emotional and physical health outcomes than victims who received no support. In addition, victims who received negative support (i.e., blaming, controlling, and diminishing) were more likely to have more negative emotional and physical health outcomes (Campbell et al., 2015). Thus, it seems that social support (or the lack thereof) is an important factor in a victim's decisions following SAV, and social support can help victims maintain a sense of self-worth (Littleton, 2010).

Media can model behaviors for viewers and influence perceptions of behaviors by showing positive and negative outcomes (Bandura, 2001). We therefore conducted research to explore how adolescent girls respond to a supportive SAV disclosure or an unsupportive SAV disclosure when compared to a control narrative that did not include any sexual assault disclosure. We specifically examined adolescent girls' reported self-efficacy to share the story they just viewed (i.e., confidence in their ability to share the story) if they were the one in the protagonist's shoes.

Method

Participants

Parents of adolescent girls (n = 77) ages 13–17 were recruited to invite their daughters to participate in this study. Most of the participants in this study were between the ages of 15 and 17 (M = 15.45; SD = 1.15) and came from 14 U.S. states. More than half of the participants were White (n = 42; 54.5%), with the next largest group being Black or African American (n = 30; 39%), followed by Asian (n = 3; 3.9%) and Hispanic or Latino (n = 3; 2.6%) participants. Participants' parents reported that the average household income was between $50,000 (28.6%) and $100,000 (29.9%), and 77.9% of parents reported having earned a bachelor's degree, advanced degree, or terminal degree.

Procedure

First, approval from the institutional review board at the primary author's university was obtained. Convenience sampling methods, social media advertising, and postings on listservs were used to recruit parents of participants. Parents read over the consent form and permitted their adolescent daughters to participate. Parents reported basic demographic information and then were instructed to leave the room and allow their daughters to come to the laptop or tablet to continue the study. Then, the participants read over the detailed assent form, agreed to participate in the study, and verified that their parents had left the room. At the end of the study, parents of participants were prompted to share the study with other parents of adolescent girls who might be interested.

Originally, the data for the current study was collected as part of a larger study that included four conditions, but this chapter focuses solely on the supportive and unsupportive SAV narratives compared to the control. Participants were randomly assigned to either view a control narrative (n = 28; i.e., no sexual assault disclosure), a supportive disclosure narrative (n = 27; i.e., where a sexual assault disclosure was met with support from others), or an unsupportive disclosure narrative (n = 22; i.e., where a sexual assault disclosure was not met with support from others).

After watching their assigned media stimuli, participants answered a series of open-ended questions to gauge their perspectives about SAV narratives in entertainment media. Then, they responded to Likert-type items about their anticipated level of self-efficacy to share their story if they were in the shoes of the protagonist. Chen et al.'s (2001) self-efficacy scale was used, which consisted of eight statements measured on a seven-point strongly disagree (1) to strongly agree (7) scale. Scores were averaged to create a scale (α = .91; M = 5.34, SD = 1.01) where higher scores indicated higher levels of anticipated self-efficacy. For more details about the measurements used, please see the Measurement Appendix.

Parents and adolescent girls then reviewed a debriefing script containing local, state, and national resources for those affected by sexual assault. During the data cleaning process, 13 cases that did not reflect an expected completion time or demonstrated failure to construct a real answer were removed from the sample.

Media stimuli

Three media stimuli were created by screen-recording, editing, and hosting media clips from Netflix and Disney+ in Canvas Studio. Stimuli were edited to remove direct portrayals of sexual violence. See Table 18.1 for summaries of the narratives. Stimuli were embedded into the online survey. The shows from which the narratives were pulled were selected, in part, because of their popularity among youth (Premack, 2018).

Qualitative data analysis procedures

This study included open-ended survey questions to best assess participants' narrative sense-making regarding the stories presented in the stimuli. Participants reflected on how they made sense of their assigned clip, including what happened to the protagonist and what would happen to

TABLE 18.1 Descriptions of media stimuli used in the study

Media Stimulus Type	Duration	Show	Synopsis of Clips Shown
Supportive Narrative	5:15	Sex Education	Aimee, a teenage girl, was sexually assaulted on a city bus by a stranger. Throughout the season, Aimee struggles with post traumatic stress disorder symptoms and finally discloses the SAV to her friends who help her make sense of what happened and face her fear of going on the bus again. The stimulus ends with Aimee facing her fears by taking the bus with her friends by her side.
Unsupportive Narrative	5:22	13 Reasons Why	Hannah was raped[a] at a party by someone she knew. Hannah failed to disclose to her friend that she was assaulted. Hannah then had a negative experience trying to talk to her school counselor about the assault. Her school counselor does not actively support her and places some blame on Hannah for causing the assault. The stimulus ends with ambiguity, leading viewers to question whether Hannah ever receives support.
Control Narrative	4:13	Doogie Kameāloha, M.D.	Lahela is a teenage girl who is a prodigy and doctor. Lahela takes her driver's test to earn her driver's license.

[a] *Rape* is defined as "Penetration, no matter how slight, of the vagina or anus with any body part or object, or oral penetration by a sex organ of another person, without the consent of the victim" (FBI, 2013). Depictions of the sexually violent act were not included in the clip.

her in the future. Following the protocol for thematic analysis identified by Braun and Clarke (2012), two independent coders made an initial pass through the data to develop first-round themes. Then, emerging themes were cross-checked for similarities and discrepancies before being condensed, revisiting the data, and finalizing the findings. Qualitative findings are noted in the results and discussion sections.

Supportive SAV disclosure narrative results

First, the results of viewing a supportive SAV disclosure narrative compared to a control narrative without any SAV disclosure were examined. An independent samples t-test was conducted to explore the differences in reported self-efficacy to share a story between those who viewed the supportive narrative and the control narrative. A Levine's test of homogeneity revealed that the variances were not significantly different, $F(2, 48) = .216$, $p = .644$. There was not a significant difference in reported self-efficacy between the supportive narrative ($M = 5.76$) and the control narrative ($M = 5.88$), $t(2, 48) = -.655$, $p = .258$. Girls who watched the supportive disclosure narrative did not feel more or less efficacious (i.e., confident in their ability) to share the protagonist's story than girls who watched the control narrative.

The qualitative responses revealed that girls exposed to the supportive SAV disclosure narrative demonstrated support for Aimee as a survivor emphasizing that Aimee could "help others who have also been sexually assaulted" in the future. Most participants in the supportive narrative condition believed that Aimee "definitely could get to a place where she is hopeful for the future" and go on to lead a fulfilling life.

Unsupportive SAV disclosure narrative results

The results of viewing an unsupportive SAV disclosure narrative compared to a control narrative without any SAV disclosure were then examined. An independent samples t-test was conducted to explore the differences in self-efficacy to share a story between those who viewed the unsupportive disclosure narrative and the control narrative. First, Levine's test of homogeneity revealed that the variances between the experiment groups were significantly different, $F(2, 53) = 6.602$, $p = .013$. There was a significant difference in reported self-efficacy to share a story between the unsupportive narrative group ($M = 4.72$) and the control group ($M = 5.88$), $t(41.078) = -4.478$, $p < .001$. Girls who watched the unsupportive disclosure narrative therefore felt significantly less efficacious (i.e., confident in their ability) to share the protagonist's story than girls who watched the control narrative that did not include an SAV narrative.

In the unsupportive narrative condition, participants engaged—perhaps consciously or subconsciously—in problematic sense-making, arguing that the main character, Hannah, "believe[d] she was assaulted even though she never said no nor told the guy to stop." the majority in the unsupportive narrative condition believed that Hannah would only be able to recover and have hope "by getting justice" in a legal case against the perpetrator.

Discussion

Both the quantitative and qualitative findings hold important implications for the role of narrative sense-making in adolescent girls' understanding of SAV. The power of narrative sense-making as a tool is reinforced by findings from extant literature (Koenig Kellas, 2017; Koenig Kellas et al., 2020), and this study extends the efficacy of narrative sense-making as a method for adolescent sense-making in SAV contexts specifically. Importantly, SAV media narratives can serve as effective vehicles for sense-making, which aligns with previous research (Riggs & Rasmussen, 2021) and affirms that narratives can serve as a practical tool for sexual assault awareness and prevention efforts.

This study found that girls who watched a supportive disclosure narrative felt equally efficacious to share their respective protagonist's story as girls who watched the control narrative, whereas girls who watched an unsupportive disclosure narrative felt significantly less efficacious to share the story than those who watched the control. As previously discussed, media models can serve "as tutors, motivators, inhibitors, disinhibitors, social prompters, emotion arousers, and shapers of values and conceptions of reality" (Bandura, 2001, p. 283). Thus, SAV narratives that model supportive SAV disclosure or unsupportive SAV disclosure could influence how adolescent girls shape their own understanding of SAV. Bandura (2001) states that people will perform behaviors if they expect to receive valuable outcomes for said behavior. In addition, fear of negative social reactions to sexual assault disclosure has been identified as a barrier to disclosure (Kennedy & Prock, 2018). It is possible that the adolescent girls in the unsupportive narrative condition did not see themselves as self-efficacious because they wanted to avoid the unwanted outcomes of disclosure as modeled in their assigned narrative. Thus, these findings have implications for those who wish to encourage self-efficacy and positive sense-making in adolescents around the topic of sexual assault.

The qualitative results revealed that adolescent girls in both the unsupportive and supportive narrative groups were able to make sense of the SAV narratives shown to them in distinct ways. The qualitative analysis results indicate that the tone and quality of a narrative can steer sense-making in helpful or harmful directions depending on what the narrative type (supportive vs. unsupportive disclosure narrative) implies about sexual assault victims, the value of social support, the stigma surrounding disclosure, and other key factors. Importantly, The CNSM's translational storytelling heuristic states that individuals engage in a collaborative sense-making process through sharing and hearing narratives (Koenig Kellas,

2017). The current findings emphasize that storytelling about sexual assault leaves critical impressions on adolescent girls' sense-making and perceptions of self-efficacy. Based on the findings in this study, we encourage further use of this theory in the context of sexual trauma narratives in digital (and) entertainment media.

These findings provide some evidence that viewing mediated narratives can act as a form of retrospective storytelling and sense-making. The findings emphasize that storytelling about sexual assault, particularly stories that are negatively framed, leaves critical impressions on adolescent girls' sense-making and perceptions of self-efficacy. Those who have a vested interest in adolescent girls' well-being, including parents, practitioners, and medical professionals, should take notice of the framing of messages within media content marketed to teenagers.

Future research should explore the influence of social support and parents' discussions with their adolescent children regarding SAV narratives in entertainment media on teen's sense-making. For example, parents who watched *13 Reasons Why* felt that they better understood the struggles their teens face during that life stage and felt more parental efficacy when talking to their teens about tough topics after exposure (Mann et al., 2022). We must acknowledge that this study would have benefited from a more robust study design that included the consideration of the effects of other demographic characteristics such as age, race and ethnicity, and education on adolescent girls' sense-making process. The protagonists in the SAV narrative stimuli were both White, relatively privileged adolescent girls, so future experiments should test racial/ethnic comparisons of SAV narrators in media in a more controlled research environment. Nevertheless, we hope this research spurs more examination of the influences of entertainment media on adolescent girls' lives, including the themes and narratives within said entertainment media, and how media might shape girls' sense-making and self-efficacy around sensitive topics like SAV.

References

Ahrens, C. E., Stansell, J., & Jennings, A. (2010). To tell or not to tell: The impact of disclosure on sexual assault survivors' recovery. *Violence and Victims, 25*(5), 631–648. https://doi.org/10.1891/0886-6708.25.5.631

Bandura, A. (2001). Social cognitive theory of mass communication. *Media Psychology, 3*(3), 265–299. https://doi.org/10.1207/S1532785XMEP0303_03

Braun, V. & Clarke, V. (2012). Thematic analysis. In H. Cooper (Ed.), *APA handbook of research methods in psychology* (Vol. 2, pp. 57–71). American Psychological Association.

Campbell, R., Greeson, M. R., Fehler-Cabral, G., & Kennedy, A. C. (2015). Pathways to help: Adolescent sexual assault victims' disclosure and help-seeking experiences. *Violence Against Women, 21*(7), 824–847. https://doi.org/10.1177/1077801215584071

Chen, G., Gully, S. M., & Eden, D. (2001). Validation of a new general self-efficacy scale. *Organizational Research Methods, 4*(62), 63–83. https://doi.org/10.1177/109442810141004

Coyne, S. M., Ward, L. M., Kroff, S. L., Davis, E. J., Holmgren, H. G., Jensen, A. C., Erickson, S. E., & Essig, L. W. (2019). Contributions of mainstream sexual media exposure to sexual attitudes, perceived peer norms, and sexual behavior: A meta-analysis. *Journal of Adolescent Health, 65*(4), 430–436. https://doi.org/10.1016/j.jadohealth.2018.11.016

Dunn, E. C., Nishimi, K., Powers, A., & Bradley, B. (2016). Is developmental timing of trauma exposure associated with depressive and post-traumatic stress disorder symptoms in adulthood? *Journal of Psychiatric Research, 84*, 119–127. https://doi.org/10.1016/j.jpsychires.2016.09.004

FBI. (2013). Rape. *FBI: Uniform Crime Reports.* https://ucr.fbi.gov/crime-in-the-u.s/2013/crime-in-the-u.s.-2013/violentcrime/rape#:~:text=The%20revised%20UCR%20definition%20of,rape%20and%20incest%20are%20excluded.

Finkelhor, D., Shattuck, A., Turner, H. A., & Hamby, S. L. (2014). The lifetime prevalence of child sexual abuse and sexual assault assessed in late adolescence. *Journal of Adolescent Health, 55*(3), 329–333. https://doi.org/10.1016/j.jadohealth.2013.12.026

Flood-Grady, E. & Koenig Kellas, J. (2019). Sense-making, socialization, and stigma: Exploring narratives told in families about mental illness. *Health Communication, 34*(6), 607–617. https://doi.org/10.1080/10410236.2018.1431016

Goodman-Brown, T. B., Edelstein, R. S., Goodman, G. S., Jones, D. P., & Gordon, D. S. (2003). Why children tell: A model of children's disclosure of sexual abuse. *Child Abuse & Neglect, 27*(5), 525–540. https://doi.org/10.1016/S0145-2134(03)00037-1

Holman, A., & Koenig Kellas, J. (2018). "Say something instead of nothing": Adolescents' perceptions of memorable conversations about sex-related topics with their parents. *Communication Monographs, 85*(3), 357–379. https://doi.org/10.1080/03637751.2018.1426870

Horstman, H. K. (2019). Young adult women's narrative resilience in relation to mother-daughter communicated narrative sense-making and well-being. *Journal of Social and Personal Relationships, 36*(4), 1146–1167. https://doi.org/10.1177/0265407518756543

Kaufman, M., & American Academy of Pediatrics Committee on Adolescence (2008). Care of the adolescent sexual assault victim. *Pediatrics, 122*(2), 462–470. https://doi.org/10.1542/peds.2008-1581

Kennedy, A. C., & Prock, K. A. (2018). "I still feel like I am not normal": A review of the role of stigma and stigmatization among female survivors of child sexual abuse, sexual assault, and intimate partner violence. *Trauma, Violence & Abuse, 19*(5), 512–527. https://doi.org/10.1177/1524838016673601

Koenig Kellas, J. K. (2017). Communicated narrative sense-making theory: Linking storytelling and well-being. In D. O. Braithwaite, E. A. Suter, & K. Floyd (eds.), *Engaging Theories in Family Communication* (2nd edition, pp. 62–74). Routledge. https://doi.org/10.4324/9781315204321

Koenig Kellas, J. K., Morgan, T., Taladay, C., Minton, M., Forte, J., & Husmann, E. (2020). Narrative connection: Applying CNSM theory's translational storytelling heuristic. *Journal of Family Communication*, 20(4), 360–376. https://doi.org/10.1080/15267431.2020.1826485

Littleton, H. L. (2010). The impact of social support and negative disclosure reactions on sexual assault victims: A cross-sectional and longitudinal investigation. *Journal of Trauma & Dissociation*, 11(2), 210–227. https://doi.org/10.1080/15299730903502946

Mann, S., Cingel, D. P., Lauricella, A. R., & Wartella, E. (2022). Parent viewership of *13 Reasons Why* and parental perceived knowledge about adolescent life: Implications for parental efficacy among parents from the United States, the United Kingdom, Brazil, and Australia/New Zealand. *Journal of Children and Media*, 16(2), 240–260. https://doi.org/10.1080/17482798.2021.1962931

McAdams, D. P. (2001). The psychology of life stories. *Review of General Psychology*, 5(2), 100–122. https://doi.org/10.1037/1089-2680.5.2.100

McElvaney, R., Greene, S., & Hogan, D. (2014). To tell or not to tell?: Factors influencing young people's informal disclosures of child sexual abuse. *Journal of Interpersonal Violence*, 29(5), 928–947. https://doi.org/10.1177/0886260513506281

Murphy, C. (2021). Out of solitary confinement: Representations of youth incarceration in young adult literature. *Children's Literature Association Quarterly*, 46(4), 401–413. https://doi.org/10.1353/chq.2021.0048

Orchowski, L. M., Untied, A. S., & Gidycz, C. A. (2013). Social reactions to disclosure of sexual victimization and adjustment among survivors of sexual assault. *Journal of Interpersonal Violence*, 28(10), 2005–2023. https://doi.org/10.1177/0886260512471085

Pajares, F. (2005). Self-efficacy during childhood and adolescence. In *Self-efficacy beliefs of adolescents* (pp. 339–367). Information Age Publishing.

Pennebaker, J. W. (2000). The effects of traumatic disclosure on physical and mental health: The values of writing and talking about upsetting events. In J. M. Violanti, D. Paton, & C. Dunning (eds.), *Posttraumatic stress intervention: Challenges, issues, and perspectives* (pp. 97–114). Charles C Thomas Publisher, Ltd.

Premack, R. (2018, June 22). *We asked 100 teens how they watch television — and the results should horrify cable companies*. Business Insider. https://www.businessinsider.com/youtube-netflix-teen-generation-z-moving-away-from-cable-2018-6

Rideout, V., Peebles, A., Mann, S., & Robb, M. B. (2022). *Common Sense census: Media use by tweens and teens, 2021*. Common Sense. https://www.commonsensemedia.org/research/the-common-sense-census-media-use-by-tweens-and-teens-2021

Riggs, R. E. & Rasmussen, E. E. (2021) The influence of video-modeled sexual assault disclosure and self-efficacy messages on sexual assault disclosure efficacy of adolescent girls. *Journal of Health Communication*, 26(6), 361–370. https://doi.org/10.1080/10810730.2021.1943729

Sandler, P. (2022, April 4). *Share of daily video content consumption among teenagers in the United States from fall 2015 to spring 2022, by platform*. Statista.

https://www-statista-com.lib-e2.lib.ttu.edu/statistics/631146/teens-video-content-platform-usa/

Schwartz, S. J., Côté, J. E., & Arnett, J. J. (2005). Identity and agency in emerging adulthood: Two developmental routes in the individualization process. *Youth & Society*, 37(2), 201–229. https://doi.org/10.1177/0044118X05275965

Seeberger, J. M., Lucas, C., Brawley, A., Groff, A., Kavanaugh, M., Yirinec, A., Moroco, A., Zhu, X., King, T. S., & Olympia, R. P. (2023). Positive and negative themes depicted in television shows targeted toward adolescents. *Clinical Pediatrics*, 62(3), 215–226. https://doi.org/10.1177/00099228221118401

Serisier, T. (2018). *Speaking out: Feminism, rape, and narrative politics*. Palgrave Macmillan.

Ullman, S. E. (2024). Aspects of selective sexual assault disclosure: Qualitative interviews with survivors and their informal supports. *Journal of Interpersonal Violence*, 39(1–2), 263–289. https://doi.org/10.1177/08862605231195808

19

ADOLESCENTS' USE OF SOCIAL MEDIA FOR SEXUAL AND REPRODUCTIVE HEALTH ADVOCACY

Jessica Fitts Willoughby, Jessica Gall Myrick, Leticia Couto, Stacey J.T. Hust, and Rebecca Ortiz

In March 2024, people in the United States could – for the first time – buy an over-the-counter oral contraceptive in stores or online (Hetter, 2024). Youth activists, along with doctors, nurses, lawyers, scientists, pharmacists, reproductive justice advocates, and public health practitioners, worked for more than a decade to make this regulatory change happen (Grossman, 2023). For example, 19-year-old Dyvia Huitron shared the barriers she faced trying to acquire birth control in a Food and Drug Administration advisory committee public hearing, saying, "we should be given the opportunity to make choices for ourselves" (Grossman, 2023). Prior to the FDA meeting, young people joined in a #FreeThePill rally in Washington, DC (URGE, 2023), and showed support for the movement online through social media posts, including use of the #FreeThePill hashtag (e.g., Bedsider, 2023).

This is just one example of teens voicing opinions, both online and through in-person demonstrations, about sexual and reproductive health topics with which they are concerned. In another example, in December 2017, more than 2,000 young people gathered in London to rally against period poverty, which is the inability for individuals to afford menstrual products, as part of the Free Periods campaign created by teen Amika George (George, 2022) that involved both online (e.g., articles and interviews) and offline (e.g., talking to politicians, giving talks) efforts. Protests and rallies are a prominent form of expressing dissent and can highlight social problems about which people collectively and publicly send a message showing their opposition (Ratliff & Hall, 2014). As of January 2020,

DOI: 10.4324/9781032648880-23

the U.K. government had given funding to schools in England to support making menstrual products available to students (George, 2022).

As these examples illustrate, teens can be prominent activists promoting changes in reproductive and sexual health policies, both online and in-person. Media can serve as a crucial resource that can help adolescents learn about reproductive health issues, find social support for dealing with these issues, and take action to address them. During adolescence, a time fraught with developmental changes and identity formation (Côté, 2009), social media is a space that teens use to project their public selves to others to communicate who they are and how they want to be perceived, also known as self-presentation (Doster, 2013). Additionally, social media serves as a space for teens to experiment with different identities and is an "accelerator in the teen identity-making process" (Doster, 2013, p. 267).

Given the important role that social media may play in teens' lives, identity formation, and self-presentation, the present work sought to 1) further our understanding of how (and how often) teens engage with controversial sexual and reproductive health topics online and 2) assess whether such digital engagement is associated with activist behaviors, specifically, engagement in rallies and demonstrations for these causes. These findings are an important step toward understanding how social media tools may be shaping modern teen activism around sexual health and reproductive rights.

Collective action, connected action, and youth

Adolescents often identify with political and social causes and integrate them into their personal identities (e.g., Martínez et al., 2012). Collective action is "the intentional action of individuals sharing a common group membership to benefit a group" (Louis, 2009, p. 727). It does not require people to be physically proximal to one another; instead, collective action focuses on the shared goals of group members in both offline and online spaces. Teens like Amika George use social media as a catalyst for collective action both online and offline. Connective action, a related but different phenomenon, is the process through which individuals come together and engage in participation and coproduction of social media content as a form of collective engagement (Vaast et al., 2017). Such efforts, like the #FreeThePill campaign, help teens coalesce around shared beliefs and goals.

Multiple factors are central in spurring people, including adolescents, to engage in collective and connective action. One of the reasons adolescents (including early, mid, and late adolescents) engage in activism is because they see it as an affirming space that celebrates aspects of their identity (Akiva et al., 2017). Social identity, for example, refers to people's sense of identification with a group of people and includes individuals' shared understandings of the meaning of group membership. According to the integrative social identity model of collective action, injustice, efficacy, and, most importantly, social identity, are key variables that predict collective action (van Zomeren et al., 2008). More specific to the context of sexual health and reproductive rights, young people also use digital media in ways that develop feminist identities in social media spaces (Gleason, 2018).

The role of media

More traditional mass media such as news tend to cover protests and dissent critically (Boyle & Schmierbach, 2009) or with a focus on violence (LeFebvre & Armstrong, 2016). However, content related to protest activity on social media tends to place more emphasis on peace (LeFebvre & Armstrong, 2016). Among those who engage in protests for politicized topics, there is greater use of the internet than more traditional media (Boyle & Schmierbach, 2009). Social media brings with it more interactive ways for people interested in similar causes to find information and connect with others. In the current context, hashtag feminism is the use of hashtags (e.g., #FreeThePill), an affordance unique to social media, to create and sustain groups of people interested in feminist-related issues, including reproductive health and efforts to address sexual justice (Myles, 2018).

The use of hashtags is just one form of potential online advocacy, however. Social media also offers other affordances that can bolster awareness and interest in causes. "Likes" and comments are also frequently used forms of expression on social media sites. Likes on social media represent the popularity of content and serve as a form of user expression that indicates appreciation (Khan, 2017). Comments, instead, allow a user to share information as part of a post. These different functionalities may serve different purposes for the people engaging with them. For example, research into likes and comments found that likes tend to be driven by brand relationships and are less impacted by self-presentation, but that shares and comments are driven by self-presentation (Swani & Labrecque, 2020).

Social media users respond to content on social media that others provide to manage their online image, and the affordances (e.g., visibility, composition of network) of different social media platforms moderate self-presentation (Hollenbaugh, 2021). It is unclear, however, how such online engagement is associated with collective action, such as participating in a demonstration or rally for a cause, around controversial topics. Based on the previously discussed literature, the following research questions guided our work:

RQ1: What behaviors are adolescents engaging in online (e.g., following content creators, sharing their own content, liking content, and using hashtags) around four potentially controversial sexual and reproductive health topics (i.e., contraceptive access, STI testing and prevention, access to menstrual products, and abortion rights)?

RQ2: Are these online behaviors associated with a greater likelihood of engagement in a rally or demonstration for the respective issue?

Method

We recruited an online convenience sample ($N = 962$) of 18- to 20-year-olds living in the United States, the United Kingdom, and Australia via the survey sampling company Prolific. We wanted to have an international sample upon which to examine these research questions and sought to collect data from countries that had recently experienced some controversy around sexual and reproductive health topics. These young adults completed an online, cross-sectional survey about their online and offline behaviors related to the four sexual and reproductive health topics. In research examining data quality in online convenience sample methods, Prolific data was found to be of higher quality, with a greater percentage of participants meaningfully responding to questions and passing attention checks, than research conducted via other platforms (i.e., MTurk, Qualtrics, and an undergraduate student research participant pool, Douglas et al., 2023). Participants were paid the equivalent of $14–16 USD (varied slightly by country) per hour for completing the survey, which took approximately 10 minutes. Recruitment messaging said that the study was about social media use and sharing their attitudes and opinions related to health topics. The consent form specified that the survey would have questions about potentially sensitive topics, including abortion and sexual health. The first author's institutional review board determined the study exempt prior to data collection.

Measures

The survey began with a series of questions about social media use and perceptions of social media sharing. Participants were then asked to indicate, on a scale from 1 (never) to 7 (very often), how often they engaged in social media behaviors (e.g., How often have you used a hashtag in support of each of the following topics?) and advocacy behaviors (e.g., How often have you participated in a rally or demonstration about the following topics?) for the following topics: contraceptive access, STI testing and prevention, access to menstrual products, and abortion rights. Item wording is available in Table 19.1 and the Measurement Appendix. Participants were also asked their perception of how controversial (1 = not at all controversial to 7 = very controversial) each issue (contraceptive access, STI testing, access to menstrual products, and abortion) was where they lived with the item "how controversial do you think the following topics are where you live?"

Participants

Participants were young adults ages 18–20 ($M = 19.1$, $SD = 0.77$) from the United States ($n = 430$, 44.7%), the United Kingdom ($n = 345$, 35.9%), and Australia ($n = 187$, 19.4%). Most participants were heterosexual ($n = 625$, 65.0%) and cisgender ($n = 906$, 94.2%). A little more than half identified as women ($n = 522$, 54.3%). Participants often identified as having a

TABLE 19.1 Percentage of participants who had engaged in the following behaviors

Item	Variable Name	Contraceptive Access	STI Testing and Prevention	Access to Menstrual Products	Abortion Rights
Liked social media content in which someone has shared their attitudes and opinions related to...	Liked else	76.2%	73.0%	76.2%	79.2%
Followed a content creator who supported...	Content creator	72.5%	67.0%	72.0%	75.3%
Shared your own attitudes and/or opinions on social media related to...	Shared own	29.1%	22.0%	28.7%	39.1%
Used a hashtag in support of	Hashtag	13.9%	12.5%	14.3%	17.7%
Participated in a rally or demonstration for	Rally	9.7%	7.5%	9.8%	16.4%

moderate income (n = 435, 45.2%), when asked on a five-point scale from very low income to very high income.

Results

In exploring RQ1, we found that, among our sample and across all topics, teens were most likely to report having "liked" social media content in which someone shared their attitudes and opinions related to the four topics (i.e., contraceptive access, STI testing and prevention, access to menstrual products, and abortion rights) when compared to engaging in other online behaviors, including following a content creator who supports the topics, sharing their own attitudes and opinions on social media, and using a hashtag in support of the topics. See Table 19.1 for all descriptives. Among online behaviors assessed, teens were least likely to report having used a hashtag in support of the topics. Our participants' involvement in rallies ranged from 7.5% for STI testing and prevention to 16.4% for abortion rights.

Across the topics, teens reported the most engagement in activism related to abortion rights. For example, while sharing their attitudes and opinions on social media ranged from 22.0% to 29.1% for the other three topics, 39.1% of teens in our sample reported having shared their attitudes and opinions on social media related to abortion rights. Teens reported the least online engagement with STI testing and prevention across all behaviors mentioned.

To address RQ2, we conducted four logistic regressions, each with participation in a rally or demonstration (related to the specific topic) as the dichotomous outcome, with the respective social media behaviors as predictor variables. For all four models (N = 962), the non-significant Hosmer–Lemeshow tests indicated good model fit. The variability explained by each model was assessed with Cox and Snell R Square and Nagelkerke R Square. See Table 19.2 for all model fit information.

In all models, gender (coded as men and other than men), income, and country of participant (coded as United States and other than United States) were not significantly associated with engagement in rallies and demonstrations for the four topics. Age was also unassociated with rallying, except for in the topic of STI testing and prevention, as older participants were more likely to have participated in a rally about the topic. The social media behaviors associated with rally engagement across all topic areas were participants sharing their own content about the topic and using a hashtag about the topic (see Table 19.3). Following a content creator for contraceptive access was also significantly associated with attending a rally about contraceptive access.

TABLE 19.2 Logistic regression model fit statistics for engaging in rally participation for sexual and reproductive health topics

	χ^2	df	p	Cox and Snell R Square	Nagelkerke R Square
Contraceptive access	177.80	9	< .001	16.9%	35.9%
STI prevention and testing	166.57	9	< .001	15.9%	38.6%
Menstrual product access	209.10	9	< .001	19.6%	41.3%
Abortion rights	191.72	9	< .001	18.1%	30.6%

TABLE 19.3 Logistic regression predicting likelihood of participating in a rally or demonstration for sexual and reproductive health topics

Contraceptive Access	B	SE	Wald	df	p	OR	95% CI	
Age	.243	.169	2.073	1	.150	1.275	0.916	1.776
Gender	.185	.296	0.393	1	.531	1.204	0.674	2.149
Income	.204	.285	0.515	1	.473	1.227	0.702	2.143
Country	.097	.159	0.371	1	.542	1.102	0.807	1.505
Local controversy	.147	.078	3.537	1	.060	1.158	0.994	1.350
Shared own	.525	.119	19.378	1	<.001	1.690	1.338	2.134
Hashtag	.785	.143	30.177	1	<.001	2.193	1.657	2.902
Liked else	-.021	.140	0.024	1	.878	0.979	0.744	1.288
Content creator	.371	.135	7.573	1	.006	1.449	1.113	1.887

STI Prevention and Testing	B	SE	Wald	df	p	OR	95% CI	
Age	.417	.195	4.555	1	.033	1.517	1.035	2.224
Gender	.104	.325	0.102	1	.749	1.109	0.587	2.097
Income	.228	.307	0.555	1	.456	1.257	0.689	2.293
Country	-.128	.183	0.486	1	.486	0.880	0.614	1.260
Local controversy	.124	.088	1.969	1	.161	1.132	0.952	1.346
Shared own	.803	.154	27.269	1	<.001	2.233	1.652	3.019
Hashtag	.694	.174	15.983	1	<.001	2.002	1.424	2.813
Liked else	-.039	.161	0.060	1	.807	0.961	0.701	1.319
Content creator	.294	.151	3.769	1	.052	1.342	0.997	1.806

Menstrual Products	B	SE	Wald	df	p	OR	95% CI	
Age	.195	.174	1.245	1	.264	1.215	0.863	1.709
Gender	.175	.316	0.306	1	.580	1.191	0.641	2.214
Income	.204	.278	0.542	1	.462	1.227	0.712	2.115

(Continued)

TABLE 19.3 (Continued)

Country	.144	.160	0.813	1	.367	1.155	0.844	1.581
Local controversy	.224	.078	8.205	1	.004	1.251	1.073	1.458
Shared own	.497	.124	16.028	1	<.001	1.643	1.289	2.096
Hashtag	.862	.148	34.026	1	<.001	2.368	1.772	3.163
Liked else	.194	.148	1.712	1	.191	1.214	0.908	1.623
Content creator	.249	.142	3.075	1	.079	1.282	0.971	1.693

Abortion Rights	*B*	*SE*	*Wald*	*df*	*p*	*OR*	95% CI	
Age	.100	.130	0.588	1	.443	1.105	0.856	1.425
Gender	-.111	.234	0.225	1	.635	0.895	0.565	1.416
Income	.243	.217	1.257	1	.262	1.275	0.834	1.949
Country	.203	.120	2.849	1	.091	1.225	0.968	1.549
Local controversy	-.087	.058	2.240	1	.134	0.917	0.818	1.027
Shared own	.369	.092	16.069	1	<.001	1.446	1.207	1.732
Hashtag	.795	.118	45.078	1	<.001	2.215	1.756	2.794
Liked else	.120	.114	1.109	1	.292	1.127	0.902	1.410
Content creator	.132	.101	1.705	1	.192	1.141	0.936	1.392

Note: Gender was coded as men = 0, other than men = 1; United States = 1, others = 0.

Discussion

In our survey data of four politically contentious reproductive and sexual health topics (i.e., contraception access, STI testing and prevention, access to menstrual products, and abortion rights) among 18- to 20-year-olds across three countries, we found that a substantial proportion of teens were using social media to engage with related content, although the amount of teens using different methods for engagement varied greatly. Approximately three-quarters of the sample reported having followed a content creator who supported the various topics. Conversely, less than a third of participants in our sample, except for in the case of abortion rights (which was 39.1%), shared their personal opinions and attitudes on social media about the different topics, with even less having reported use of a hashtag. As adolescence is a time of identity formation (Côté, 2009) and social media can be influential while teens are developing their identities and provide a space in which teens may experiment with different identities (Doster, 2013), such behaviors could be examples of topics that adolescents care about and for which they want to present an image of concern. The adolescents we surveyed were less engaged online with STI testing and prevention than the other topics. Although STIs are prevalent among young adults, this, in part, could be due to the stigma often associated with STIs (e.g., NASEM, 2021). Although abortion is also often stigmatized, different types of stigma exist around sexual and reproductive health topics (e.g., Hall et al., 2018). Adolescents may have less interest in more prominently engaging with the topic of STIs than other sexual and reproductive health-related topics.

Among the online behaviors assessed, we found that some forms of online engagement were associated with the likelihood of having participated in a rally for the cause. Among participants, sharing their attitudes about the topics online and using hashtags in support of the topics were both associated with greater likelihood of attending rallies and demonstrations. However, liking the content of others was not associated with a greater likelihood of attending a rally or demonstration. This difference could be due to the different social media functions of sharing one's views versus liking others' statements. Likes on social media express an appreciation for content, and they may indicate popularity of the content (Khan, 2017). However, sharing involves a conscious decision to make the post available to one's network (Khan, 2017). In marketing research, comments and sharing, as opposed to liking and other reactions, may be driven by self-presentation (Swani & Labrecque, 2020). According to the integrative social identity model of collective action, social identity is a primary driver of engagement in collective action (van Zomeren et al., 2008).

Our findings that hashtag use was associated with a greater likelihood of mobilizing for rallies and demonstrations also provide evidence that there is a link between online social media activity and advocacy actions. Hashtags specifically offer the affordance of aggregating similar content and making it easier to find (Clark, 2016), which can then bring attention to issues and "create momentum for digital feminist activism" (Myles, 2018, p. 510). This momentum, in turn, allows people to voice concerns and be heard. The combination of identifying oneself while connecting with others who also care about that topic may be another factor that more closely links adolescents' identities with a social movement, which in turn might motivate them to get out the door and engage in public displays of this newly strengthened identity as someone who cares about sexual health and reproductive rights. It can make them feel part of a group, which teens are desperately looking for in their identity formation. Adolescents actively seek peer approval, and even though they may hesitate to take social risks for fear of peer exclusion, they will engage in said behaviors if they are endorsed by their peers (Tomova et al., 2021).

Although the findings of which online behaviors were associated with rally participation were consistent across the four topic areas, only among contraceptive access was following a content creator who supported the topic associated with a greater likelihood of participating in a related rally. This could be due to the specific content area, as the amount of social media posts that discuss contraceptive access increased from 2006 to 2019, with this content becoming increasingly positive, especially about long-acting reversible contraceptive methods (Merz et al., 2021). Although for STI testing and prevention and menstrual product access, following a content creator was significant-adjacent ($p = .052$ for STI prevention and treatment, $p = .079$ for menstrual product access) in its relationship to attending a rally, following a content creator for abortion rights was clearly non-significant in its association with participating in a rally or demonstration for the topic. This may highlight that for some topics, especially one that, in this case, could be considered the most highly politicized, the online action of following others does not translate directly to behaviors. There may be religious, cultural, and political considerations that also affect abortion-related public advocacy in ways that are not as influential for other topics. Notably, there is an increasing amount of misinformation and disinformation about abortion circulated online (Pagoto et al., 2023). This means that following content creators could mean that people are exposed to greater misinformation that demotivates them from participating in public events.

As with any research, the limitations of the work must be considered. Although our data spanned three countries, the data were cross-sectional, thus causation cannot be determined; our findings are limited to the countries and cultural experiences of those within them. Also, our use of a convenience sampling method means that prevalence data cannot be generalized from the findings. Lastly, although we can speculate on some of the underlying reasons for differences based on theory and research, we did not specifically examine causal pathways that could further explain engagement in behaviors. Future work would benefit from taking a longitudinal approach to further examine engagement in such behaviors over time, ideally across various stages of development, so that research can further our understanding among early, mid, and late adolescents.

Conclusion

Our survey of 18- to 20-year-olds across three countries found that many teens have actively engaged with content on social media about contraceptive access, STI testing and prevention, menstrual product access, and abortion rights. Having shared their attitudes and opinions and having used a hashtag in support of these topics were all online actions associated with an increased likelihood of having attended a rally or demonstration for the related cause. For contraceptive access rallies, having followed a content creator who supported contraceptive access was also associated with an increased likelihood of attending a rally. These behaviors were more strongly associated with rally or demonstration participation across the topic areas than were demographic factors, such as gender, age, income, or living in an area in which the topic was controversial. Future research is needed to address these important ongoing issues at the intersection of digital media, adolescent development, advocacy, and media effects.

References

Akiva, T., Carey, R. L., Cross, A. B., Delale-O'Connor, L., Brown, M. R. (2017). Reasons youth engage in activism programs: Social justice or sanctuary. *Journal of Applied Developmental Psychology*, 53, 20–30. https://doi.org/10.1016/j.appdev.2017.08.005

Bedsider [@Bedsider]. (2023, May 2). Yup – no prescription or ID required, just put it in your cart and check out #TnxBrithControl #FreeThePill. [Tweet]. *Twitter*. https://twitter.com/Bedsider/status/1786131168611500528

Boyle, M. P., & Schmierbach, M. (2009). Media use and protest: The role of mainstream and alternative media use in predicting traditional and protest participation. *Communication Quarterly*, 57(1), 1–17. https://doi.org/10.1080/01463370802662424

Douglas, B. D., Ewell, P. J., & Brauer, M. (2023). Data quality in online human-subjects research: Comparisons between MTurk, Prolific, CloudResearch, Qualtrics, and SONA. *PLOS One*. https://doi.org/10.1371/journal.pone.0279720

Doster, L. (2013). Millennial teens design and redesign themselves in online social networks. *Journal of Consumer Behaviour*, 12(4), 267–279.

Clark, R. (2016). 'Hope in a hashtag': The discursive activism of #WhyIStayed. *Feminist Media Studies*, 16(5), 788–804. https://doi.org/10.1080/14680777.2016.1138235

Côté, J. E. (2009). Identity formation and self-development in adolescence. *Handbook of Adolescent Psychology*, 1(3), 266–304.

Gleason, B. (2018). Adolescents becoming feminist on Twitter: New literacies practices, commitments, and identity work. *Journal of Adolescent & Adult Literacy*, 62(3), 281–289.

George, A. (2022, May 25). How I helped convince the U.K. to provide free period products in schools. *The Washington Post*. https://www.washingtonpost.com/lifestyle/2022/05/25/amika-george-period-poverty-activism/

Grossman, D. (2023, July 19). The victory for over-the-counter birth control pills is just the beginning. *The New York Times*. https://www.nytimes.com/2023/07/19/opinion/birth-control-pills-opill-over-the-counter.html

Hall, K. S., Morhe, E., Manu, A., Harris, L. H., Ela, E., Loll, D., ... & Dalton, V. K. (2018). Factors associated with sexual and reproductive health stigma among adolescent girls in Ghana. *PloS One*, 13(4), e0195163. https://doi.org/10.1371/journal.pone.0195163

Hetter, K. (2024, March 5). Who can take the newly available over-the-counter birth control pill? *CNN*. https://www.cnn.com/2024/03/05/health/birth-control-opill-pregnancy-wellness/index.html#:~:text=The%20first%20oral%20contraceptive%20approved,for%20a%20three%2Dmonth%20supply.

Hollenbaugh, E. E. (2021). Self-Presentation in social media: Review and research opportunities. *Review of Communication Research*, 9, 80–98. https://doi.

org/10.12840/ISSN.2255-4165.027; https://www.researchgate.net/publication/ 354616146_Self-Presentation_in_Social_Media_Review_and_Research_ Opportunities

Khan, M. L. (2017). Social media engagement: What motivates user participation and consumption on YouTube? *Computers in Human Behavior*, 66, 236–247. https://doi.org/10.1016/j.chb.2016.09.024

LeFebvre, R. K., & Armstrong, C. (2016). Grievance-based social movement mobilization in the #Ferguson Twitter storm. *New Media & Society*, 20(1): 8–28. https://doi.org/10.1177/1461444816644697

Louis, W. R. (2009). Collective action—and then what? *Journal of Social Issues*, 65(4): 727–748. https://doi.org/10.1111/j.1540-4560.2009.01623.x

Martínez, M. L., Peñaloza, P., & Valenzuela, C. (2012). Civic commitment in young activists: Emergent processes in the development of personal and collective identity. *Journal of Adolescence*, 35(3): 474–484. https://doi.org/10.1016/j. adolescence.2011.11.006

Merz, A. A., Gutiérrez-Sacristán, A, Bartz, D, Williams, N.E., Ojo, A., Schaefer, K. M., Huang, M., Li, C. Y., Sandoval, R. S., Ye, S, Cathcart, A. M., Starosta, A., & Avillach, P. (2021). Population attitudes toward contraceptive methods over time on a social media platform. *American Journal of Obstetrics and Gynecology*, 224(6), 597.e1–597.e14. https://doi.org/10.1016/j.ajog.2020.11.042

Myles, D. (2018). 'Anne goes rogue for abortion rights!': Hashtag feminism and the polyphonic nature of activist discourse. *New Media & Society*, 21(2), 507–527. https://doi.org/10.1177/1461444818800242

NASEM National Academies of Sciences, Engineering and Medicine. (2021). *Sexually transmitted infections: Adopting a sexual health paradigm*. The National Academies Press. https://doi.org/10/17226/25955

Pagoto, S. L., Palmer, L., & Horwitz-Willis, N. (2023). The next infodemic: Abortion misinformation. *Journal of Medical Internet Research*, 25, e42582. https://doi.org/10.2196/42582

Ratliff, T. N., & Hall, L. L. (2014). Practicing the art of dissent: Toward a typology of protest activity in the United States. *Humanity & Society*, 38(3): 268–294. https://doi.org/10.1177/0160597614537796

Swani, K., & Labrecque, L. I. (2020). Like, comment, or share? Self-presentation vs. brand relationships as drivers of social media engagement choices. *Marketing Letters*, 31(2), 279–298. https://doi.org/10.1007/s11002-020-09518-8

Tomova, L., Andrews, J.L., & Blakemore, S. (2021). The importance of belonging and the avoidance of social risk taking in adolescence. *Developmental Review*, 61https://doi.org/10.1016/j.dr.2021.100981

URGE Unite for Reproductive and Gender Equity [@urge_org]. (2023, May 13). Come with URGE to last week's Free The Pill Rally, hosted by @free_the_pill! This year's rally was particularly special because. *Instagram*. https://www. instagram.com/urge_org/reel/CsL3VXtgWCL/

Vaast, E., Safadi, H., Lapointe, L., & Negoita, B. (2017). Social media affordances for connective action: An examination of microblogging use during the Gulf of Mexico oil spill. *MIS Quarterly*, 41(4), 1179–1206.

van Zomeren, M., Postmes, T., & Spears, R. (2008). Toward an integrative social identity model of collective action: A quantitative research synthesis of three socio-psychological perspectives. *Psychological Bulletin*, 134(4), 504–535. https://doi.org/10.1037/0033-2909.134.4.504

20

SECTION 3 COMMENTARY

Adolescents as Engagers and Creators: Opportunities for Media Education and Advocacy

Jessica Fitts Willoughby, Rebecca Ortiz, and Stacey J.T. Hust

Teens frequently engage in the creation of media (e.g., Guerrero-Pico et al., 2019) and can improve the effectiveness of sexual health-related digital interventions through their involvement in content creation (Bennett et al., 2023; Martin et al., 2020). The chapters in this section highlighted ways in which adolescents engage with and learn from media about sexual health. Specifically, in Chapter 17, Dodson and Scull found that media literacy skills, which can be developed through media literacy education interventions, can impact sexual health behaviors and reduce potential harmful effects of media on sexual health. Their results across multiple samples and studies showed the benefits of improving media literacy among adolescents and the potential for media literacy to serve concurrently as a sexual health educator. They found that, although intervention effects varied on media processing skills among the different adolescent samples, there were consistent results in the areas of sexual health communication self-efficacy (e.g., confidence in talking to a partner about contraception) and in contraception use self-efficacy (e.g., confidence in their ability to use contraception correctly). Additionally, the intervention also had an influence on risky sexual behaviors among young adults (the only sample with which the outcome was examined), such that 18- and 19-year-olds reported less sexual activity with someone not tested for an STI or with an unknown STI status.

Although the authors have many important takeaways from their work, a major point was that media literacy education shows promise for sexual health education across developmental stages and format, given the various ages that the interventions were tested with and that some

DOI: 10.4324/9781032648880-24

interventions were digital and others in person. In a review of literature that examined adolescents' perceptions of school-based sexual health education, Corcoran et al. (2020) identified that adolescents often found sexual health education lacking and wanted honest and comprehensive content delivered in nonjudgmental ways by credible professionals in a comfortable environment. Although more work needs to be done to further examine differences in modality preferences for media literacy education interventions, as discussed in the Dodson and Scull chapter, the method shows great promise as a potential sexual health education opportunity for youth.

When not provided with adequate sexual health information, young people often seek out such information, oftentimes by going online. In Chapter 18, Zelaya and colleagues highlighted how digital media, in particular the internet, has not served young people in meeting their sexual health information needs. They found that young adults felt the information they accessed online as teens lacked actionable guidance, authentic depictions of anatomy, and diverse and inclusive content. They suggested that those working to enhance sexual health education should focus on content that not only acknowledges potential harms but also focuses on discussions of pleasure, emotional intimacy, and social contexts, which aligns with other definitions of sexual health (e.g., NASEM, 2021; World Health Organization, 2024) and encouragement from researchers to adopt a sexual health paradigm that promotes sexual health as a part of overall wellbeing (e.g., Boyer et al., 2021). Zelaya and colleagues also highlighted the importance of the inclusion of sexual and gender minorities and reflecting information that may speak to their experiences, harkening back to the importance of representation (as discussed in the commentary for the first section of this book; Chapter 8).

Even when not seeking out sexual health content, media serves as a sexual health educator. Riggs and colleagues (Chapter 19) found that teens' self-efficacy in sharing the protagonist's story after exposure to a supportive narrative surrounding sexual assault victimization did not significantly differ from those in a control condition. However, teens who viewed the unsupportive sexual assault victimization narrative reported less self-efficacy to share the protagonist's story than participants who were in the control group. These findings highlight the role that narratives can play in teens' behaviors related to sexual violence and support previous research (e.g., Hust et al., 2015).

Even when teens watch content that could be considered harmful (e.g., sexual violence), there are opportunities in which learning can take place, given the modeling that occurs. Teens who watch programming in which sexual assault victims are not supported, which may be common given that mass media often portray stereotypes related to sexual assault (i.e., rape myths), show skepticism toward survivors, and favor perpetrators (e.g., Aroustamian, 2020), may be less likely to speak out in such situations, given that efficacy is often associated with behavior (e.g., Theory of Planned Behavior, Ajzen, 1991). However, when one sees a character speak out about a sexual assault experience and receive support, it may reduce potential fears about disclosing one's own experiences, should such experiences occur. Entertainment education, which is the imbedding of educational content in entertaining media (Singhal & Rogers, 2012), is often guided by social cognitive theory (Bandura, 2001), which posits that how characters who model behaviors are either rewarded or punished for those behaviors may impact how those watching enact the behaviors in their own lives. Sexual assault entertainment education content developed based on social cognitive theory as well as the inclusion of other theoretical frameworks (i.e., social norms) has been found to lead to greater self-efficacy related to sexual assault prevention for young adults when compared to viewing content not associated with sexual assault (Hust et al., 2017). Riggs and colleagues' work has similar implications, highlighting that the specific actions portrayed in a narrative and how they are experienced by the characters can be seen as modeled behaviors that may impact teens' confidence in sharing similar stories.

In contrast to the previous chapters that focused more on individual effects, Willoughby et al. (Chapter 20) showcased some of the ways in which teens engage with digital media for sexual health advocacy. The researchers found that teens in three countries engaged in the online sharing of content around the following four topics of interest: contraceptive access, STI prevention and treatment, menstrual product access, and abortion rights. Online engagement was associated with attending rallies and demonstrations about the issues, and teens used strategies to share information that was likely pertinent to their identity development.

Although media literacy had its own chapter in this section, we would also be remiss if we did not further discuss the role media literacy likely plays in all the different areas discussed in this section. Given that one of the main concerns about sexual health information online is trust and credibility (e.g., Farrugia et al., 2021), skills in media literacy could also play a valuable role for adolescents in interpreting the plethora of content to which adolescents are exposed when seeking online. Dodson and Scull (Chapter 17) found positive effects on sexual health knowledge through their media literacy education intervention. Additionally, when young adults are reflective about the media with which they engage, including how they act as a source of content, they also consider how the content that they present on social media may impact others (Willoughby & Couto,

2024). Media literacy may be a powerful tool for adolescents, as it gives them the agency to act with a greater understanding of the impact of media on them but also the impact on others that they may have based on the content they share and create online.

As with all research, the studies described here were not without limitations. Cross-sectional designs (e.g., Zelaya et al., Chapter 18; Willoughby et al., Chapter 20) and the largely United States samples limit the conclusions in terms of generalizability, although they are in line with much of the research being conducted in the field overall (see Willoughby et al., Chapter 1). Riggs and colleagues' use of a single message design limits our ability to extend the findings beyond the specific stimuli used in the experiment. And Dodson and Scull's work is limited by the single media literacy program described, as we cannot speak more broadly to media literacy development in other ways outside the intervention described in the case study. Regardless, the research provides further insight into how media can be used as sources of education and advocacy for teens and areas for future research.

Future efforts would benefit from increased consideration of the role media literacy plays in all aspects of media interpretation among adolescents, as well as content creation and dissemination. The specific presentations of media examined in Riggs and colleagues' work helped to remind us of the importance of continuing to move beyond mere effects studies to understanding how specific portrayals are received by youth and may impact relevant constructs, and especially how the impact of viewing this content may shift as the content to which youth are exposed shifts. Zelaya and colleagues' work highlighted the importance of continuing to refine how sexual health information is provided and how adolescents are aided in the curation of the plethora of sexual-related content available online. Lastly, Willoughby and colleagues' chapter highlighted how we need to continue focusing on research that considers teens as both content creators and consumers. Overall, this section provided insights into the ways adolescents engage with and create content, and the implications their engagement and creation have in relation to their sexual health education and decision-making.

References

Ajzen, I. (1991). The theory of planned behavior. *Organizational Behavior and Human Decision Processes*, *50*(2), 179–211. https://doi.org/10.1016/0749-5978(91)90020-T

Aroustamian, C. (2020). Time's up: Recognising sexual violence as a public policy issue: A qualitative content analysis of sexual violence cases in the media. *Aggression and Violent Behavior*, *50*, 101341. https://doi.org/10.1016/j.avb.2019.101341

Bandura, A. (2001). Social cognitive theory: An agentic perspective. *Annual Review of Psychology, 52*(1), 1–26.

Bennett, C., Musa, M. K., Carrier, J., Edwards, D., Gillen, E., Sydor, A., ... & Kelly, D. (2023). The barriers and facilitators to young people's engagement with bidirectional digital sexual health interventions: a mixed methods systematic review. *BMC Digital Health, 1*(1), 30. https://doi.org/10.1186/s44247-023-00030-3

Boyer, C. B., Agênor, M., Willoughby, J. F., Mead, A., Geller, A., Yang, S., Prado, G. J., & Guilamo-Ramos, V. (2021). A renewed call to action for addressing the alarming rising rates of sexually transmitted infections in U.S. adolescents and young adults. *Journal of Adolescent Health, 69*(2), 189–191. https://doi.org/10.1016/j.jadohealth.2021.05.002

Corcoran, J. L., Davies, S. L., Knight, C. C., Lanzi, R. G., Li, P., & Ladores, S. L. (2020). Adolescents' perceptions of sexual health education programs: An integrative review. *Journal of Adolescence, 84*, 96–112. https://doi.org/10.1016/j.adolescence.2020.07.014

Farrugia, A., Waling, A., Pienaar, K., & Fraser, S. (2021). The "be all and end all"? Young people, online sexual health information, science and skepticism. *Qualitative Health Research, 31*(11), 2097–2110. https://doi.org/10.1177/10497323211003543

Guerrero-Pico, M., Masanet, M. J., & Scolari, C. A. (2019). Toward a typology of young produsers: Teenagers' transmedia skills, media production, and narrative and aesthetic appreciation. *New Media & Society, 21*(2), 336–353. https://doi.org/10.1177/1461444818796464

Hust, S. J.T., Adams, P. M., Willoughby, J. F., Ren, C., Lei, M., Ran, W., & Marett, E. G. (2017). The entertainment-education strategy in sexual assault prevention: A comparison of theoretical foundations and a test of effectiveness in a college campus setting. *Journal of Health Communication, 22*(9), 721–731. https://doi.org/10.1080/10810730.2017.1343877

Hust, S. J. T., Marett, E., Lei, M., Ren, C. & Ran, W. (2015). *Law & Order, CSI,* and *NCIS*: The association between exposure to crime drama franchises, rape myth acceptance and sexual consent negotiation behaviors among college students. *Journal of Health Communication, 20*, 1369–1381. http://doi.org/10.1080/10810730.2015.1018615

Martin, P., Cousin, L., Gottot, S., Bourmaud, A., de La Rochebrochard, E., & Alberti, C. (2020). Participatory interventions for sexual health promotion for adolescents and young adults on the internet: Systematic review. *Journal of Medical Internet Research, 22*(7), e15378. https://doi.org/10.2196/15378

NASEM National Academies of Sciences, Engineering and Medicine. (2021). *Sexually transmitted infections: Adopting a sexual health paradigm.* The National Academies Press. https://doi.org/10/17226/25955

Singhal, A., & Rogers, E. (2012). *Entertainment-education: A communication strategy for social change.* Routledge.

Willoughby, J. F. & Couto, L. (2024). Social media and fitness content: A mixed methods study of ecological momentary assessment as an intervention. Presented at the Kentucky Conference on Health Communication, Lexington, KY.

World Health Organization. (2024). *Sexual health.* https://www.who.int/health-topics/sexual-health#tab=tab_1

CONCLUSION

21

ENVISIONING THE FUTURE OF TEENS, SEX, AND MEDIA RESEARCH

Stacey J.T. Hust, Jessica Fitts Willoughby, and Rebecca Ortiz

The chapters in this book provided a robust examination of how adolescents incorporate and are impacted by sexual media content. However, the chapters also revealed that there is still much left to learn about how adolescents incorporate media content into their romantic and sexual lives, and how exposure to and engagement with sexual media content affects their well-being. Further understanding of these topics will help scholars, parents, educators, policymakers, and health practitioners address some of the more pressing issues facing adolescents today (e.g., unplanned pregnancy, sexually transmitted infections, identity development, and sexual violence), especially as they play out in ever-evolving media environments.

Despite the critical need for this research, our state of the field review (Willoughby et al., Chapter 1) revealed that fewer papers were published about teens, sex, and media recently than in previous years; in 2023, researchers published more than 50% fewer articles ($n = 14$) than in 2014 ($n = 31$). The results of our researcher survey provide potential insight into why we see this decline (Ortiz et al., Chapter 2).

The researchers in our survey wrote about the challenges they experienced during the research process (e.g., recruitment and IRB approval) and a lack of available funding as significant barriers to completing their research. Some also shared that they faced criticism and verbal attacks when conducting research related to media and adolescents' romantic and sexual lives. Some even reported that they left the field because of these challenges. Additionally, when we solicited proposals for the current book, a few potential authors declined to participate for fear that they would face professional

DOI: 10.4324/9781032648880-26

consequences (i.e., tenure denial and/or loss of employment). The challenges experienced by researchers are sometimes too much to overcome.

Such challenges are likely due, at least in part, to the stigmas associated with adolescent sexual activity, which are then amplified in certain socio-political environments, such as U.S. states that ban abortions (e.g., Idaho or Texas) or countries that pass anti-LGBTQ+ legislation (e.g., Uganda). As researchers ourselves who can relate to some of these challenges, we find it disconcerting (although unsurprising) that faculty and other scholars fear personal and professional repercussions for doing such important work, especially given the importance of the research and how it often benefits some of the most vulnerable people in our societies.

As indicated by our state of the field review and researcher survey, the decline in publications and challenges researchers face conducting this research, resulting in some leaving the field, reveal cautionary implications for the future of research on teens, sex, and media. One of the pioneers of the field, Jane D. Brown, Ph.D., began investigating adolescents, sex, and media in the 1980s. She continued actively researching and mentoring others in this area until she retired from the University of North Carolina at Chapel Hill in 2012, but it may be difficult for other scholars to similarly dedicate their careers to this area of research. Having junior scholars join the field and bring new ideas is highly beneficial, but for a body of research to develop and grow, we also need established researchers with robust experience and insight. As a researcher gains experience in the field, they can systematically build and expand upon past work, furthering understanding of how communication and media are related to teens' relationship development and sexual health. They can also mentor junior researchers through the barriers and challenges of doing this work, helping set them up for future success and longevity. As outlined in Chapter 2 (Ortiz et al.), we call on institutions and funders to help in reducing these barriers to ensure researchers can succeed, and the adolescents served by this research can benefit.

Despite the challenges the field faces, we are optimistic and excited about the committed researchers who shared in our survey that they are highly motivated to continue their research, as they acknowledged the positive impact their work can have on young people. We are also proud of the work published within this book, which will contribute uniquely to the field and help move it forward in important ways. We, therefore, conclude this book by highlighting some of the key insights gleaned from the research and provide reflections for how researchers can continue to strengthen and enhance research about teens, sex, and media.

Conducting inclusive research

Some of the researchers from our survey acknowledged that they faced challenges specific to recruiting diverse and/or representative samples, in particular youth who identify as LGBTQ+ (Ortiz et al., Chapter 2). Despite these challenges, many of the researchers in this book were able to recruit incredibly diverse samples regarding nationality, gender identity, and sexual orientation. For example, 52.4% of the youth surveyed by Dajches and colleagues (Chapter 7) identified as LGBQ+, which allowed the researchers to examine and find differences by sexual identity in the ways in which celebrity idolization affects teen girls' sexual self-concept, whereas, as they noted, most past research had focused on heterosexual girls.

The teens interviewed by Hust and colleagues (Chapter 3) and the older adolescents who participated in L'Pree Corsbie-Massay's (Chapter 5) and Mares and Chen's (Chapter 6) studies also highlighted how media rarely or inadequately portray LGBTQ+ people. As we learned from their research, such symbolic annihilation of gender and sexual identity diversity in the media has significant consequences for teens who may turn to the media to learn about their or others' identities, especially in the absence of in-person examples. Mares and Chen's study (Chapter 6), in particular, showcased the importance of these portrayals, as they can create opportunities for LGBTQ teens to gauge others' (in this study, parents') reactions and support of their identities when watching media portrayals together. The teens thankfully reported more positive than negative outcomes, but the negative were deeply concerning as some of the comments included insinuations of violence (e.g., when a transgender teen reported that their parent said "he would 'beat the shit' out of his child if they thought they were trans") and emotional turmoil experienced by the teens (e.g., when a bisexual teen said "I watched for my mother's reaction while watching, and she seemed ... almost disgusted. It made me feel terrible about myself."). These results reveal an urgent need for more research and efforts dedicated to supporting teens in their identity exploration and development, especially LGBTQ+ teens, to ensure their health and well-being.

Media have a powerful role to play in identity development, as teens in these studies highlighted several positive outcomes, such as using media portrayals to better understand diverse gender and sexual identities (theirs or others) and to foster fruitful conversations with others. These studies provide a strong foundation for future research that explores ways in which the media can be used to promote the acceptance of diverse youth populations, including gender and sexual minorities.

Furthering scientific rigor

As was identified by researchers in our survey and our state of the field review, research on teens, sex, and media can continue to benefit from increased scientific rigor. This includes continuing to move beyond cross-sectional designs and convenience samples and pushing for more representative samples and longitudinal (i.e., over time) designs when possible. However, structural barriers in the academic systems, where most of the researchers who published research from 2013 to 2023 are employed, may negatively impact researchers' abilities to do so.

It is important for researchers to push back against or circumnavigate some of the barriers that limit their abilities to engage in rigorous methodologies. For example, the continued heightening of expectations around the quantity of research needed for successful tenure reviews/promotion may not allow researchers time to develop the relationships needed for longitudinal research with adolescent audiences. Additionally, lack of time and resources may make obtaining funds to secure representative and generalizable samples difficult. In the long term, it would be beneficial to change these structures so that expectations for tenure adjust to the requirements of conducting sensitive research with adolescents. It is also important that additional funding opportunities are made available to help researchers tackle these issues. In the interim, however, opportunities for collaboration could be productive. Researchers, for example, may look to collaborate with existing public health data collection efforts to reach more generalizable samples by bringing stronger media exposure measures to such collaborations.

Improved measurement as an area for further development

The field would also benefit from improvements in measurement of media usage and exposure. Ward called for researchers to move beyond measuring mere exposure to media content and instead focus more on the ways in which adolescents engage and internalize media (Ward, 2016), especially since measurement of media exposure has often been fraught with errors, such as inaccurate recall and recognition biases (Niederdeppe, 2014), which are further amplified in digital communications (Niederdeppe, 2016).

Many of the authors in this book extended existing research by following Ward's suggestion. For example, L'Pree Corsbie-Massay (Chapter 5), Ward et al. (Chapter 10), and Zelaya et al. (Chapter 17) focused on how participants retroactively remembered experiences with media content or asked participants to move beyond media to which they were exposed to identify the ways in which they engaged with the content. Hust et al. (Chapter 3) and Riggs et al. (Chapter 18) asked youth about their perceptions of media content and found that youth make sense of media in myriad ways, often viewing content through existing gender and sexual scripts (e.g., Kim et al., 2007). Additional chapters considered adolescents as producers of media content instead of simply passive recipients and examined factors associated with that content production (Van Ouytsel et al., Chapter 11; Densley et al., Chapter 12; Martinez-Bacaicoa et al., Chapter 13; Willoughby et al., Chapter 19). Continuing to think about the different ways in which teens engage with, create, and use media will further enhance the field by providing more nuanced perspectives on effects, allowing for a greater understanding of *how* and *why* the effects occurred instead of just noting that they exist.

Additionally, research in this field can continue to benefit by examining media effects in person-specific ways. Valkenburg et al. (2024), for example, found differences in person-specific effects of social media on adolescent well-being, such that some adolescents were negatively impacted, while others experienced positive impact. Their work highlighted that the ways teens react to and are impacted by media vary, and work that relies on overall findings may miss these individual or group differences.

Newer approaches to measurement are also needed given that teen media diets can vary significantly. Although research that examines the effects of specific media programs or content can be beneficial, we urge researchers to continue recognizing that media effects rarely occur in isolation. Like many of us, teens often engage in media multitasking, quickly switching between media or using more than one form of media at a time (Ettinger & Cohen, 2020; Kaiser Family Foundation, 2013). Measuring exactly what teens are exposed to can become an impossible task, in part because of their highly personalized media diets (e.g., algorithms on social media vary greatly). Talking to teens more qualitatively, such as using open-ended, teen-informed techniques, instead of more structured and inflexible quantitative questions, may therefore not only be preferable but necessary. Additionally, measurements that allow for a greater understanding of the perceptions of content taken over repeated time points could be valuable at influencing our understanding of person-specific effects (e.g., ecological momentary assessment or intensive longitudinal designs, Valkenburg et al., 2024).

Given the frequency with which teens' use of media continues to adapt and change, there is also great benefit to engaging more directly with teens in the research and measurement process. As reported in Chapter 2 (Ortiz et al.), researchers in the field felt that it was important to involve young people more actively in research, as they often have important ideas for furthering our understanding of media effects on themselves and their peers. Adolescent steering committees, where teens serve as advisory boards for research studies, are one beneficial way for increased understanding and agency for adolescents, for whom this work is meant to benefit.

Developing (and testing) measurements that work in various cultures is also important as media environments become increasingly global. As Hust and colleagues (Chapter 4) found in their research where they used the heterosexual script scale (Seabrook et al., 2016) with teens in six different countries, measurement scales developed and used primarily with adolescents in one country may be applicable to adolescents elsewhere and further our understanding of differences across cultures and geographic regions.

Also, further testing and refinement of scales and constructs in general before use can help the field by providing stronger measurement overall. For example, the technology-facilitated sexual violence scale used by Martínez-Bacaicoa et al. (2024) (Chapter 13) with Spanish teens can benefit other researchers by offering a tested scale that may be applicable to teens in many different cultures. To assist in these efforts, we have included a measurement appendix in this book so that scholars can easily and readily access scales used successfully by the book's researchers.

Acknowledging the increasingly digital lives of teens

Today's youth are living increasingly digital lives, and as argued in Hust et al. (Chapter 14), the digital landscape increasingly includes sexual content. It is important then for scholars to identify how teens define and operationalize their digital sexual lives. Multiple studies in this book considered youths' online interactions, with three chapters specifically considering teens' sexting. We applaud the authors of these chapters for using specific language (e.g., image-based sexting) to describe the actions of their participants as not all sexting behaviors are the same. As these chapters indicate, online sexual activity can include consensual behaviors, such as text- or image-based sexting, but it also includes nonconsensual behaviors, such as sextortion and digital sexual harassment. We encourage researchers to continue to refine the operationalization and standardization of digital sexual activity so that we can more precisely understand teens' sexual lives online. For example, researchers studying sexual violence may want to include the host of behaviors identified by Martinez-Bacaicoa and colleagues (Chapter 13) as they consider the many ways teens encounter sexual violence in digital spaces in their daily lives.

We acknowledge, however, that we are from a different generation than the teens included in these studies. They are digital natives living in a profoundly different environment from many who are scholars today. The lead editor of this book, for example, can remember sending her first email during her first year at college, whereas many of the youth today are texting friends in elementary school. In another example, some adults are concerned about the digital permanence of the internet, especially as it relates to image-based sexting, in part because they worry that such images may be used maliciously against the teens at some point (e.g., Cleveland Clinic, 2024). Some teens, however, may not be concerned about such permanence and may consider ways in which they can share such images without disclosing their identity (e.g., not showing their faces or other identifying marks). Given the generational differences between scholars and teen participants, it is important for researchers to involve teens in all aspects of their research, which may include having them participate in a steering committee to review study protocols and questionnaires and asking them to help interpret study results.

The role of media literacy and sex positivity

Relatedly, teens today are not simply passive viewers of media but are active engagers and content creators. The work by Zelaya et al. (Chapter 17) and Willoughby et al. (Chapter 20) considered this by asking about the information young people had previously sought out or shared, respectively. Willoughby et al., for example, found that teens are using social media to advocate for sexual and reproductive health-related causes, which is associated with their advocacy (i.e., rally and demonstration attendance).

Furthering teens' understanding of the role they play in media effects, in part through media literacy education, can help adolescents as they navigate the often-changing digital media environment. Media literacy is a person's ability to access, analyze, create, and act using different forms of communication (National Association for Media Literacy Education, 2024). As discussed by Dodson and Scull (Chapter 16), media literacy can be a valuable tool for adolescents to better understand the impact of media messages on their sexual health and how they learn from media, especially in the absence of comprehensive sex education. Sexual health education, particularly in the United States, in which Dodson and Scull's work was conducted, varies greatly between states and cities (Planned Parenthood, 2024). Media literacy may help fill that gap so teens can more accurately make sense of the sexual content to which they are exposed.

Additionally, parents can play a role by discussing or reacting to media content, possibly influencing their children's views related to sexual health and relationships (e.g., Mares et al., Chapter 6). However, this can be difficult as the effects are only as good as the quality of media that spur conversations and the conversations that parents are having with teens. Campaigns that encourage parents in their efforts to communicate with teens about sexual health in a positive way could help increase efficacy in having such conversations (Willoughby & Guilamo-Ramos, 2022). In general, parents, including some of those with religious backgrounds who are often thought to support abstinence-only sex education, report that they want their teens to have sexual health knowledge, and they want such information to be provided in a sex positive way (e.g., Dent & Maloney, 2017).

Researchers have called for the adoption of a paradigm in which sexual health and sexuality are recognized as essential to overall health and well-being, and that conversations among parents, schools, and communities about these topics are encouraged (Boyer et al., 2021). However, conversations and research about teen sexuality have often taken a negative framework, focused on the risks, shame, and stigmas of sexuality, partly in hopes that it will influence young people to refrain from engaging in sexual activity, but, instead, often results in teens feeling shame or confusion about their sexuality (e.g., Hunt, 2023; Waling et al., 2020). Sex positivity, however, embraces the idea that sex is a normal and healthy part of the human experience and that discussions of consent, safety, and respect are considered alongside young people's sexual agency, interests, and desires (Ivanski & Kohut, 2017).

Taking a sex-positive approach to research on teens, sex, and media is vital for moving the field forward. This is also in line with the information and approach that young people have requested (Zelaya et al., Chapter 17). The current framework of shame, stigma, and taboo is part of what keeps the current structural barriers, as discussed earlier in this chapter, in place, making this research not just challenging but sometimes impossible to do. When these fears and stigmas rule people's decisions about whether to engage with or support teen sexuality and media research, it results in a lesser likelihood that researchers will meet the goals we set forth above. It limits researchers' abilities to conduct rigorous scientific research with improved measurement, diverse and inclusive samples, and to involve youth in those efforts.

A sex-positive lens instead allows for a nuanced understanding of how teens interact with and interpret sexual content in the media they consume. Rather than assuming all sexual media exposure is inherently harmful, sex-positive research explores both the positive and negative effects, as well as how media representations shape teens' sexual attitudes, beliefs, and behaviors. As researchers, we must continue to drive this narrative home so we can do this important research and help inform efforts to improve young people's lives.

References

Boyer, C. B., Agênor, M., Willoughby, J. F., Mead, A., Geller, A., Yang, S., Prado, G. J., & Guilamo-Ramos, V. (2021). A renewed call to action for addressing the alarming rising rates of sexually transmitted infections in U.S. adolescents and young adults. *Journal of Adolescent Health*, 69(2): 189–191.

Cleveland Clinic (2024, May 9). *Sexting: The risks and how to talk to your children about it.* https://health.clevelandclinic.org/how-to-guide-your-children-through-the-minefield-of-sexting

Dent, L., & Maloney, P. (2017). Evangelical Christian parents' attitudes toward abstinence-based sex education: 'I want my kids to have great sex!' *Sex Education*, 17(2), 149–164. https://doi.org/10.1080/14681811.2016.1256281

Ettinger, K., & Cohen, A. (2020). Patterns of multitasking behaviours of adolescents in digital environments. *Education and Information Technologies*, 25, 623–645. https://doi.org/10.1007/s10639-019-09982-4

Kaiser Family Foundation. (2013). *Media multitasking among American youth: Prevalence, predictors and pairings.* https://www.kff.org/wp-content/uploads/2013/01/7593.pdf

Kim J. L., Sorsoli C. L., Collins K., Zylbergold B. A., Schooler D., Tolman D. L. (2007). From sex to sexuality: Exposing the heterosexual script on primetime network television. *The Journal of Sex Research*, 44(2), 145–157. https://doi.org/10.1080/00224490701263660

Hunt, C. (2023). 'They were trying to scare us': College students' retrospective accounts of school-based sex education. *Sex Education*, 23(4), 464–477. https://doi.org/10.1080/14681811.2022.2062592

Ivanski, C., & Kohut, T. (2017). Exploring definitions of sex positivity through thematic analysis. *The Canadian Journal of Human Sexuality*, 26(3), 216–225. https://doi.org/10.3138/cjhs.2017-0017

Martínez-Bacaicoa, J., Sorrel, M. A., & Gámez-Guadix, M. (2024). Development and validation of technology-facilitated sexual violence perpetration and victimization scales among adults. *Assessment*, 10731911241229575. https://doi.org/10.1177/10731911241229575

National Association for Media Literacy Education. (2024). *What is media literacy?* https://namle.org/resources/media-literacy-defined/

Niederdeppe, J. (2014). Conceptual, empirical, and practical issues in developing valid measures of public communication campaign exposure. *Communication Methods and Measures*, 8(2), 138–161. https://doi.org/10.1080/19312458.2014.903391

Niederdeppe, J. (2016). Meeting the challenge of measuring communication exposure in the digital age. *Communication Methods and Measures*, 10(2–3), 170–172. https://doi.org/10.1080/19312458.2016.1150970

Planned Parenthood. (2024). *What's the state of sex education in the U.S.?* https://www.plannedparenthood.org/learn/for-educators/whats-state-sex-education-us#:~:text=Federal%20&%20State%20Policy%20Related%20to,or%20which%20school%20they%20attend.

Seabrook, R. C., Ward, L. M., Reed, L., Manago, A., Giaccardi, S., & Lippman, J. R. (2016). Our scripted sexuality: The development and validation of a measure of the heterosexual script and its relation to television consumption. *Emerging Adulthood*, 4(5), 338–355. https://doi.org/10.1177/2167696815623686

Valkenburg, P. M., Beyens, I., Bij de Vaate, N., Janssen, L., & van der Wal, A. (2024). Person-specific media effects. In T. Araujo, & P. Neijens (Eds.), *Communication Research into the Digital Society: Fundamental Insights from the Amsterdam School of Communication Research* (pp. 233–245). Amsterdam University Press. https://doi.org/10.2307/jj.11895525.17

Waling, A., Bellamy, R., Ezer, P., Kerr, L., Lucke, J., & Fisher, C. (2020). 'It's kinda bad, honestly': Australian students' experiences of relationships and sexuality education. *Health Education Research*, 35(6), 538–552. https://doi.org/10.1093/her/cyaa032

Ward, L. M. (2016). Media and sexualization: State of empirical research, 1995–2015. *The Journal of Sex Research*, 53(4–5), 560–577. https://doi.org/10.1080/00224499.2016.1142496

Willoughby, J. F. & Guilamo-Ramos, V. (2022). Designing a parent-based national health communication campaign to support adolescent sexual health. *Journal of Adolescent Health*, 70(1), 12–15. https://doi.org/10.1016/j.jadohealth.2021.09.023

MEASUREMENT APPENDIX

In this appendix, readers can find all measurements or references to published scales as used in the studies described throughout the text. Measurements created and adapted by the authors in this book can be found in full form, whereas scales that have been previously published include sample items and the citation to the publication with the original scale. Several chapters of this book (e.g., Chapter 1, Chapter 2, and Chapter 21) highlighted the need for rigor in the communication field, and we believe scholarship can be improved with transparency and access to materials. It is our hope that this appendix assists future scholars in furthering the communication field. If the reader chooses to use one of these measurements, we ask that they cite the author that developed the scale in question. If the author is one of the authors of this book, please cite their chapter in your work.

Chapter 4: Mediated Identities: A Qualitative Exploration of How Adolescents from Six Countries Make Sense of Gender Identity and Sexual Orientation in Media

The Heterosexual Script Scale (Seabrook et al., 2016)
Anchor points: 1 = Strongly Disagree; 6 = Strongly Agree
Sample item(s): Guys like to play the field and shouldn't be expected to stay with one partner for too long.
Note: In the chapter, the authors used a 1 to 5 scale.

Chapter 7: Girls Just Wanna ... Figure Out Their Sexuality: Exploring the Links Between Celebrity Idolization and U.S. Adolescent Girls' Sexual Self-Concept

Celebrity Idolization Scale (Engle & Kasser, 2005)
Anchor points: 1 = Strongly Disagree; 5 = Strongly Agree
Sample item(s):

- I own accessories (such as t-shirts, bed sheets, bracelets, key chains, buttons, hats, etc.) that show that I'm their fan.
- I vote for _____ on television award shows such as the Music Video Awards to show my support for them.
- I'm one of the first to know any new information or rumors about _____.

Sexual Anxiety Subscale From the Sexual Self-Concept Questionnaire (Snell, 1998)
Anchor points: 1 = Not at all characteristic of me; 5 = Very characteristic of me
Sample item(s):

- Thinking about the sexual aspects of my life often leaves me with an uneasy feeling.
- I feel nervous when I think about the sexual aspects of my life.
- I anticipate that in the future, the sexual aspects of my life will be frustrating.

Sexual Self-Esteem Subscale From the Sexual Self-Concept Questionnaire (Snell, 1998)
Anchor points: 1 = Not at all characteristic of me; 5 = Very characteristic of me
Sample item(s):

- I am pleased with how I handle my own sexual tendencies and behaviors.
- I have positive feelings about the way I approach my own sexual needs and desires.
- I feel good about the way I express my own sexual needs and desires.

Situational Self-Efficacy and Resistive Self-Efficacy Scales (Rostosky et al., 2008)
Anchor points: 1 = I definitely can't do this; 5 = I can definitely do this
Sample item(s):

- How sure are you that you would be able to tell someone that you didn't want to go somewhere because of what might happen sexually?
- How sure are you that you would be able to say "no" to having sexual intercourse with someone whom you want to date again?

Enjoyment of Sexualization Scale (Liss et al., 2011)
Anchor points: 1 = Strongly Disagree; 7 = Strongly Agree
Sample item(s):

- I love to feel sexy.
- I like showing off my body.
- When I wear revealing clothing, I feel sexy and in control.

Chapter 10: What Becomes of the Pretty Princess? Childhood Princess Engagement and Women's Gender and Relationship Conceptions in Late Adolescence

Modified From Wishful Identification Scale (Hoffner & Buchanan, 2005)
Anchor points: 1 = Strongly Disagree; 5 = Strongly Agree
Sample item(s):

- [This princess] is the sort of person I wanted to be like myself.
- Sometimes I wished I could be more like [this princess].
- [This princess] was someone I wanted to emulate.
- I'd wanted to do the kinds of things [this princess] did in the movie featuring her.
- I would have NEVER wanted to act the way [the princess] did in the movie featuring her.

Modified From Parasocial Interaction Scale (Rubin & Perse, 1987)
Anchor points: 1 = Strongly Disagree; 5 = Strongly Agree
Sample item(s):

- [This princess] made me feel comfortable, as if I was with a friend.
- I saw [this princess] as a natural, down-to-earth person.
- After watching the movie with [this princess], I looked forward to seeing her in other platforms, such as books, games, and toys.
- I looked forward to seeing [this princess] again by re-watching the movie featuring her.
- If [this princess] was in another Disney movie, I would have watched that movie too.

- I found [this princess] to be attractive.
- I wanted to meet [this princess] in person.
- I would pretend that [this princess] was my friend in real life.

Surveillance Subscale of the Objectified Body Consciousness Scale (McKinley & Hyde, *1996*)
Anchor points: 1 = Strongly Disagree; 6 = Strongly Agree
Item(s):

- I rarely think about how I look. (reverse-coded)
- I often worry whether the clothes I am wearing make me look good.

Body Shame Subscale of the Objectified Body Consciousness Scale (McKinley & Hyde, 1996)
Anchor points: 1 = Strongly Disagree; 6 = Strongly Agree
Sample item(s): I feel like I must be a bad person when I don't look as good as I could.

Body Appreciation Scale-2 (Tylka & Wood-Barcalow, 2015)
Anchor points: 1 = Never; 5= Always
Sample item(s):

- I respect my body.
- I appreciate the different and unique characteristics of my body.

Enjoyment of Sexualization Scale (Liss et al., 2011)
Anchor points: 1 = Strongly Disagree; 6 = Strongly Agree
Sample item(s):

- I like showing off my body.
- I love to feel sexy.

Self-Sexualization Behavior Scale-Women (Smolak et al., 2014)
Anchor points: 1 = Never; 5= Always
Stem: Please indicate how often you do each of the following things specifically in order to look sexy
Sample item(s):

- Wear high heels.
- Wear perfume/scents.

The Sexual Appeal Self-Worth Scale (Gordon & Ward, 2000)
Anchor points: -3 = Ugh, I would feel worthless; +3 Wow! I would feel really great about myself
Stem: How would you feel about yourself if
Sample item(s):

- You were asked to be a model in a calendar featuring college students.
- You gained 30 pounds.

The Heterosexual Script Scale (Seabrook et al., 2016)
Anchor points: 1 = Strongly Disagree; 6 = Strongly Agree
Sample item(s): Guys like to play the field and shouldn't be expected to stay with one partner for too long.

Romantic Beliefs Scale (Sprecher & Metts, 1989)
Anchor points: 1 = Strongly Disagree; 7 = Strongly Agree
Sample item(s): I believe if another person and I love each other, we can overcome any differences and problems that may arise.

Romantic Relationships Subscale of the Conformity to Feminine Norms Inventory – Short Form
(Parent & Moradi, 2010)
Anchor points: 1 = Strongly Disagree; 5 = Strongly Agree
Sample item(s):

- Being in a romantic relationship is important.
- Having a romantic relationship is essential in life.

Chapter 11: Image-Based Sexting and Sexual Abuse Experiences among Early Adolescents

Sexting behaviors
Anchor points: 1 = never to 5 = very often
Item(s):

- I have sent a sexually explicit picture (naked or half-naked) of myself to someone through the Internet or mobile phone.
- Someone sent a sexually explicit picture of themselves to me.
- I have asked someone to send a sexually explicit picture (naked or half-naked) of themselves to me.

Image-based sexual abuse, adapted (Gámez-Guadix et al., 2018)
Anchor points: 1 = never to 5 = very often
Sample item(s):

- Someone persisted or pressured me to send a sexually explicit picture of myself to that person.
- I have forwarded a sexually explicit picture of someone or showed it to other people, or posted it online without having permission to do so.

Adult online sexual objectification, adapted (Gámez-Guadix et al., 2018)
Anchor points: 1 = never to 5 = very often
Sample item(s):

- An adult asked me to send sexually explicit images or videos of myself through the Internet or the mobile phone.
- An adult sent me sexually explicit images or videos of themselves though the Internet or the mobile phone.

Chapter 12: Peers Versus Pixels: Teen Sexting as Influenced by Peer Norms and Pornography Use

Pornography use
Question: How often do you consume pornography?
Response options: 1 = "Never", 2 = "Less than once a month", 3 = "1-3 times a month", 4 = "Once a week", 5 = "Several times a week", 6 = "Every day" and 7 = "Several times a day"

Sexting behaviors – sending, receiving, and soliciting
Questions:

- (Sending) In the last 12 months, how often have you sent a sexually explicit image or message of yourself by cell phone?
- (Receiving) In the last 12 months, how often have you received a sexually explicit image or message of someone else by cell phone?
- (Soliciting) In the last 12 months, how often have you asked someone to send you a sexually explicit image or message of themselves by cell phone?

Response options: 1 = "Never", 2 = "Less than once a month", 3 = "1-3 times a month", 4 = "Once a week", 5 = "Several times a week", 6 = "Every day" and 7 = "Several times a day"

Peer Norms – Close Descriptive Norms and Distal Descriptive Norms
Questions:

- (Close descriptive norms) How often do you think your guy friends are sexting?
- (Close descriptive norms) How often do you think your girl friends are sexting?
- (Distal descriptive norms) How often do you think the typical guy your age is sexting?
- (Distal descriptive norms) How often do you think the typical girl your age is sexting?

Response options: 1 = "Never", 2 = "Less than once a month", 3 = "1-3 times a month", 4 = "Once a week", 5 = "Several times a week", 6 = "Every day" and 7 = "Several times a day"

Peer Norms – Close Injunctive Norms
Response options: 1 = "Strongly disapprove", 2 = "Disapprove", 3 = "Neutral", 4 = "Approve", 5 = "Strongly approve"

Item(s):

- How do you think most of your friends would feel about you sexting?
- How do you think your best friend would feel about you sexting?
- How do you think your boyfriend/girlfriend would feel about you sexting? If you don't have a boyfriend/girlfriend, imagine that you do.

Peer Norms – Distal Injunctive Norms
Response options: 1 = "Strongly disapprove", 2 = "Disapprove", 3 = "Neutral", 4 = "Approve", 5 = "Strongly approve"

Item(s):

- How do you think most girls your age would feel about you sexting?
- How do you think most guys your age would feel about you sexting?

Chapter 13: Technology-Facilitated Sexual Violence Among Adolescents: Prevalence, Age, and Gender Differences, Changes Over Time, and Mental Health Outcomes

Technology-Facilitated Sexual Violence Victimization Scales – Gender-Based Violence
Anchor points: 0 = "Never", 1 = "1 or 2 times", 2 = "3 or 4 times" and 3 = "5 times or more"
Stem: Through the Internet (in forums, chats, video games, etc.) or cell phone (e.g., social networks), during the last 12 months, how often have the following things happened to you?
Item(s):

- Someone has insulted you because you were a girl. *
- Someone has made fun of you because you were a girl. *
- Someone has humiliated, belittled, or made you feel inferior because you were a girl. *
- Someone has discriminated against you or excluded you from an online group, forum, or chat because you were a girl. *
- Someone has insulted you because you were a boy. **
- Someone has made fun of you because you were a boy. **
- Someone has humiliated, belittled, or made you feel inferior because you were a boy. **
- Someone has discriminated against you or excluded you from an online group, forum, or chat because you were a boy. **

Note: *These items were only answered by girl participants; **these items were only answered by boy participants

Technology-Facilitated Sexual Violence Victimization Scales (Gender role-based violence, sexual orientation-based violence, digital sexual harassment, nonconsensual sexting, and coercion)
Anchor points: 0 = "Never", 1 = "1 or 2 times", 2 = "3 or 4 times" and 3 = "5 times or more"
Stem: Through the Internet (in forums, chats, video games, etc.) or cell phone (e.g., social networks), during the last 12 months, how often have the following things happened to you?

Gender role-based violence
Item(s):

- Someone has insulted you for looking "too masculine" or doing "boys' things." *

- Someone has made fun of you for looking "too masculine" or doing "boys' things." *
- Someone has humiliated, belittled, or made you feel inferior for looking "too masculine" or doing "boys' things." *
- Someone has discriminated against you or excluded you from an online group, forum, or chat for looking "too masculine" or doing "boys' things." *
- Someone has insulted you for looking "too feminine" or doing "girls' things." **
- Someone has made fun of you for looking "too feminine" or doing "girls' things." **
- Someone has humiliated, belittled, or made you feel inferior for looking "too feminine" or doing "girls' things." **
- Someone has discriminated against you or excluded you from an online group, forum, or chat for looking "too feminine" or doing "girls' things." **

Note: *These items were only answered by girl participants; **these items were only answered by boy participants

Sexual orientation-based violence
Item(s):

- Someone has insulted you because of your sexual orientation.
- Someone has made fun of you because of your sexual orientation.
- Someone has humiliated, belittled, or made you feel inferior because of your sexual orientation.
- Someone has discriminated against you or excluded you from an online group, forum, or chat because of your sexual orientation.

Digital sexual harassment
Item(s):

- Someone has directed sexual comments at you that have made you feel bad.
- Someone has asked you sexual questions that have made you feel bad.
- Someone has insisted you send sexual photos or videos that have made you feel bad.

Nonconsensual sexting
Item(s):

- Someone has shown someone else sexual content of you (photos or videos) without your consent.

- Someone has posted sexual content of you (photos or videos) on the Internet without your consent.
- Someone has forwarded sexual content of you (photos or videos) without your consent.

Sexual coercion
Item(s):

- You have been threatened with showing a sexual image of yourself to another person.
- You have been threatened with publishing a sexual image of you on the Internet.
- You have been threatened with sending on the Internet a sexual image of you.

Chapter 18: Adolescent Girls' Sense-Making about Sexual Assault Victimization After Exposure to a Sexual Assault Narrative in Media

Self-Efficacy for sharing a story, adapted (Chen et al., 2001)
Anchor points: 1 = Strongly Disagree; 7 = Strongly Agree
Stem: Please imagine again that you were in [Aimee's/Lahela's/Hannah's/the teenagers'] shoes. If you were in [Aimee's/Lahela's/Hannah's/the teenagers'] shoes, how would you feel if you were to share your story with a friend or family member?
Item(s):

- I would be able to achieve the goal of sharing my story.
- I would be certain that I could accomplish the difficult task of sharing my story.
- I could share my story because it is important to me.
- I could succeed at sharing my story if I set my mind to it.
- I would be able to successfully overcome challenges related to sharing my story.
- I would be confident that I could share my story.
- I could share my story well, compared to other people.
- I could share my story even when things are tough.
- I would be able to achieve the goal of sharing my story.
- I would be certain that I could accomplish the difficult task of sharing my story.

Chapter 19: Adolescents' Use of Social Media for Sexual and Reproductive Health Advocacy

Online and other advocacy behaviors
Anchor points: 1 (never) to 7 (very often)
Item(s):

- Liked social media content in which someone has shared their attitudes and opinions related to...
- Followed a content creator who supported...
- Shared your own attitudes and/or opinions on social media related to...
- Used a hashtag in support of
- Participated in a rally or demonstration for

References

Chen, G., Gully, S. M., & Eden, D.. (2001). Validation of a new general self-efficacy scale. *Organizational Research Methods*, 4(62), 63–83. https://doi.org/10.1177/109442810141004

Engle, Y., & Kasser, T. (2005). Why do adolescent girls idolize male celebrities? *Journal of Adolescent Research*, 20(2), 263–283. https://doi.org/10.1177/0743558404273117

Gámez-Guadix, M., De Santisteban, P., & Alcazar, M. Á. (2018). The construction and psychometric properties of the questionnaire for online sexual solicitation and interaction of minors with adults. *Sexual Abuse*, 30(8), 975–991. https://doi.org/10.1177/1079063217724766

Gordon, M. K., & Ward, L. M. (2000, March). I'm beautiful, therefore I'm worthy: Assessing associations between media use and adolescents' self-worth. Paper presented at the Biennial Meeting of the Society for Research on Adolescence, Chicago, IL.

Hoffner, C., & Buchanan, M. (2005). Young adults' wishful identification with television characters: The role of perceived similarity and character attributes. *Media Psychology*, 7(4), 325–351. https://doi.org/10.1207/S1532785XMEP0704_2

Liss, M., Erchull, M. J., & Ramsey, L. R. (2011). Empowering or oppressing? Development and exploration of the Enjoyment of Sexualization Scale. *Personality and Social Psychology Bulletin*, 37(1), 55–68. https://doi.org/10.1177/0146167210386119

McKinley, N. M., & Hyde, J. S. (1996). The objectified body consciousness scale: Development and validation. *Psychology of Women Quarterly*, 20(2), 181–215. https://doi.org/10.1111/j.1471-6402.1996.tb00467.x

Parent, M., & Moradi, B. (2010). Confirmatory factor analysis of the Conformity to Feminine Norms Inventory and development of an abbreviated version: The CFNI-45. *Psychology of Women Quarterly*, 34(1), 97–109. https://doi.org/10.1111/j.1471-6402.2009.01545

Rostosky, S. S., Dekhtyar, O., Cupp, P. K., & Anderman, E. M. (2008). Sexual self-concept and sexual self-efficacy in adolescents: A possible clue to promoting sexual health? *The Journal of Sex Research*, 45(3), 277–286. https://doi.org/10.1080/00224490802204480

Rubin, A., & Perse, E. (1987). Audience activity and soap opera involvement: A uses and effects investigation. *Human Communication Research*, 14(2), 246–268. https://doi.org/10.1111/j.1468-2958.1987.tb00129.x

Seabrook, R. C., Ward, L. M., Reed, L., Manago, A., Giaccardi, S., & Lippman, J. R. (2016). Our scripted sexuality: The development and validation of a measure of the heterosexual script and its relation to television consumption. *Emerging Adulthood*, 4(5), 338–355. https://doi.org/10.1177/2167696815623686

Smolak, L., Murnen, S. K., & Myers, T. A. (2014). Sexualizing the self: What college women and men think about and do to be "sexy." *Psychology of Women Quarterly*, 38(3), 379–397. https://doi.org/10.1177/0361684314524168

Snell, W. E. (1998). The multidimensional sexual self-concept questionnaire. In C.M. Davis, W. L. Yarber, R. Bauserman, G. Schreer, S. L. Davis (Eds.), *Handbook of sexuality-related measures* (pp. 521–524). Sage.

Sprecher, S., & Metts, S. (1989). Development of the 'Romantic Beliefs Scale' and examination of the effects of gender and gender-role orientation. *Journal of Social and Personal Relationships*, 6(4), 387–411. https://doi.org/10.1177/0265407589064001

Tylka, T., & Wood-Barcalow, N. (2015). The Body Appreciation Scale-2: Item refinement and psychometric evaluation. *Body Image*, 12, 53–67. https://doi.org/10.1016/j.bodyim.2014.09.006

INDEX

Pages in *italics* refer to figures and pages in **bold** refer to tables.